PRAISE FOR THIS BOOK

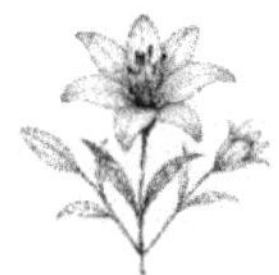

When so many people have questions about mental illness, Elizabeth Arce takes us into the world of someone who has been there—and overcame. *One of Two Ways* will not only educate you about the reality of mental illness, but it will also inspire you to overcome and lead others to do the same. The end result is that we get the healing and God gets the glory!

—RANDY D. GARCIA, Radio Show Host,
Executive Pastor, Three:16 Church

Elizabeth Arce is not only a *gifted* writer, but she is also an *anointed* one. This Biblically grounded book is a must-read for anyone dealing with fear, anxiety, and depression. Through her lived experiences, Elizabeth takes you through her own journey while providing her learned wisdom along the way. Her ability to relate to her audience on a deep level, while clearly and effectively communicating biblical insights, is astounding. I strongly suggest reading this book yourself and also passing it on to others when the Spirit moves you.

—RANDALL SEAN GARCIA, Lead Pastor, Three:16 Church

One of Two Ways

Finding Balance in Mental Illness Through a Relationship with Christ

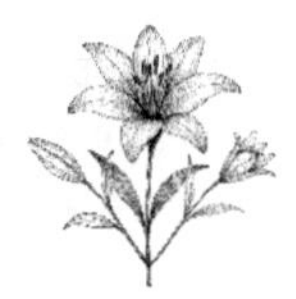

ELIZABETH ARCE

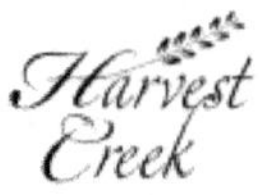

Harvest Creek Publishing & Design
www.harvestcreek.net

One of Two Ways: A Testimony—1st ed.

ISBN 978-1-961641-50-1

Printed in the United States

CONTENTS

DEDICATION

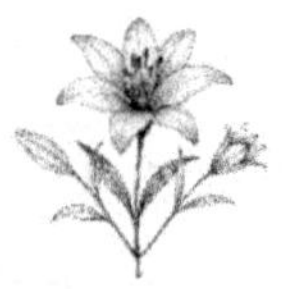

This book is dedicated to everyone
who has contemplated suicide.
As you stand at the edge of the cliff of death,
ready to jump, turn around, and see Christ!
His arms are open to you.
Run to Him and choose life!

ACKNOWLEDGMENTS

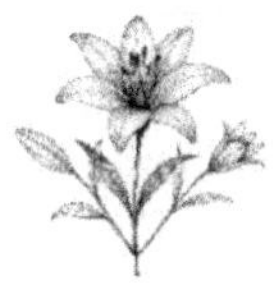

To my parents, Jerry and Beth:
Thank you for raising me to know Jesus.

To my husband, Jose:
Thank you for loving me as Christ loves His church.

To my son, Geraldo:
Thank you for your precious smile.

To my friend, Janice:
Thank you for growing and changing with me.

To Three16 Church:
Thank you for making a disciple out of me.

PREFACE

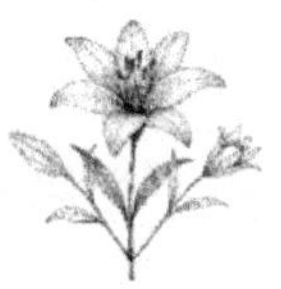

For many years, from early childhood to adulthood, I allowed anxiety and depression to influence and oppress me. I've suffered and struggled through more of my life than I have not, stumbling into sin and tripping over imperfection continuously. Yet, through it all, God's plan to deliver me unfolded. The proof of His transformative love, offered generously and graciously, is precisely what leads me to share my experiences with mental illness so candidly.

Reflecting on the darkness that once consumed me has been painful, yet healing. My healing has been so profound that I cannot, in good conscience, keep it to myself. I do not endeavor to tout a deluded sense of self-righteousness, but simply to help others change and be changed. Today I am free of sin, confusion, and disorder thanks to the gift of salvation and the divine direction that it extends.

Once I was lost, but now I am found, by grace through faith in Jesus Christ, my Lord and Savior. It is by His direction that I wrote this book, and by His will that you are reading it. This story is not my life's work, but God's work in specific and relevant seasons throughout my life. Detailed in hindsight, these slices of time showcase God's constant faithfulness despite my own erratic unfaithfulness.

I proclaim and declare this only to honor and glorify The One True God, the living God of the Holy Bible, who is sufficient in all things. Whatever I lack is found in Him, through reading His Word and being in His presence. His power is perfected in my weakness. One of these so-called "weaknesses" is that I do not have an impressive list of accomplishments or accreditations that qualify me to talk on this matter. According to the world's standards, I am a nobody. Yet, God has called me to action undeterred.

Continuing in the vein of transparency, my first answer to God's call was an emphatic "No." It seemed to me, as an extremely introverted and private person, particularly torturous to be tasked with publicly recording and analyzing my failures. However, the more I learn about the God who died for me, the more I believe in His undying love. What finally drew me to say "Yes" was not obligation or guilt, but an overwhelming desire to love Him back.

Those who say "salvation is free, but discipleship is costly" are right. My flesh fights me every step of the way, my mind wraps itself in dizzying loops, and my heart trembles in the face of the unknown. Still, the Holy Spirit cries out from within me, "Let go of control and let me lead." Releasing my own aspirations and ambitions to make room for God's plans has been challenging, but I trust it is a worthy sacrifice. My prayer is that God will also do for you what He has done for me, many times over.

—ELIZABETH ARCE

INTRODUCTION

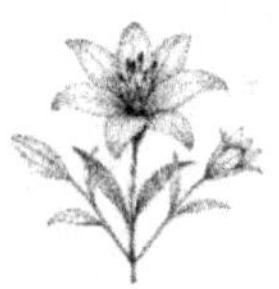

The title of this work, *One of Two Ways*, came to me in a dream, describing the reality in which we are bound. In terms of eternity, God gives us the opportunity, through free will, to choose life or death. Accept salvation and receive the promise of Heaven. Reject salvation and receive the punishment of Hell. There is no third option. In fact, despite the thousands of religions and belief systems in existence, there is only one way to get to Heaven and receive eternal life.

Jesus answered,
"I am the way and the truth and the life.
No one comes to the Father [in Heaven]
except through me."
John 14:6, NIV [EMPHASIS ADDED]

Eternity aside, there is also a lesser-known, parallel choice—a daily one—to make between life and death. He asks us to follow Him in obedience along a path of truth and grace. Yet, we so often turn back to the comforts of our rebellion, falsehood, and self-determination. For many years, despite being spiritually alive in Him, I did not follow Him and so chose the downward spiral of death.

Mental illness has been present in the world for as long as anyone can distinguish, just like physical illness. It has been documented in ancient societies and debated likewise by scholars. More importantly, it has been a consistent source of suffering (and, of course, death) for many people. Unlike the sores of leprosy or the jaundice of yellow fever, disorders of the mind cannot be so plainly seen. Because of this, they have often been misunderstood and mistreated despite increased efforts in the modern world to understand and treat them.

One etiology, or root cause, cannot be assigned to all conditions, nor the individuals experiencing said conditions, other than that we live in a broken world. Some are born with a genetic predisposition. A few are burdened by inescapable conflict or poverty. Others are subject to violence, abuse, or trauma. Many have lost spiritual purpose, or perhaps never found it in the first place. Most sufferers experience a particular combination of these generalities either in succession or simultaneously, culminating in an unmanageable amount of stress.

These afflictions result from controllable and/or uncontrollable human failure in an imperfect reality. Each of these people, male and female, old and young, rich and poor, struggles differently. But they are all inextricably linked by the truth. The perfect God who created them according to unique plans and purposes wants to be reunited with them in love, despite their inherent and often willful brokenness.

Arguably the most recognizable Bible passage, hailing from the book of John, explains our undeniable need for a savior and God's unmatched desire to save humanity.

For God so loved the world that he gave his one and only
Son, that whoever believes in him shall not perish
but have eternal life. For God did not send his Son
into the world to condemn the world,
but to save the world through him.

JOHN 3:16–17, NIV

Regardless of the diverse manners in which we struggle—with or without mental illness—God's saving grace is, and will always be, sufficient.

It's difficult to prove my adamant faith that having a relationship with the Creator is sufficient to navigate all of life's challenges, including mental illness; it might be easier to prove that the world's limited understanding does *not* present the best choice. Many times, including for me, it isn't sufficient at all. Throughout human history, attempts to innovate and improve have only led to the need for more innovation and improvement.

Instead of these advantages and privileges bringing great prosperity on earth, there has been a massive influx of physical, mental, and spiritual issues. Utopia by human means is truly unattainable. Ease and convenience are not the answer. The stressors of the future will inevitably replace the stressors of the past. A world of infinite and unpredictable problems requires one constant and independent solution. The solution is knowing Jesus Christ, who is God.

Many would argue that I have little to no evidence to support the unbelievable claim that God can solve unsolvable problems. I have no proof other than my own testimony of transformation and, of course, the testimonies of countless others. Most don't believe that God can cure incurable illness. Yet, the miracles of the Old and New Testaments are truly alive and well. The evidence lives in me. I was mentally disturbed to the point of dysfunction. And now I am not.

My healing experience is like the woman described in Mark, whose body was stuck in a broken menstrual cycle. The verses say:

And a woman was there who had been subject to bleeding for twelve years. She had suffered a great deal

[cont'd next page]

under the care of many doctors and had spent all she had,
yet instead of getting better she grew worse.
MARK 5:25–26, NIV

Undoubtedly, this relentless condition caused her tremendous physical and emotional pain.

This woman's life centered on her bleeding. For twelve years, she bled, and that blood, according to Jewish law, made her ceremonially unclean. She could not touch or be touched by anyone, nor was she able to go to the temple. She likely lived isolated from her community, including any friends and family she might have had. This bleeding separated her from meaningful relationships, intentional purpose, and even formal fellowship with God.

As anyone in such a position of suffering would, including myself, she sought relief. Yet the efforts she made to put an end to her misery did not help. No medicine, treatment, or doctor's care could stop her bleeding or ease her pain. These attempts were not just unsuccessful, as proven by her worsening condition, but they were harmful. She looked for answers from the world and the wisdom of man, but found nothing true or lasting.

My life centered on anxiety, depression, and countless other mental illness variations. For many years, I, too, suffered through life, unsure of how long it would take and how far I'd have to go to be clean and free.

I was ruled and confined by the effects of my ailment. Reliance on doctors and medicine only left me disappointed and confused. Ultimately, I had questions and problems that only God could answer and solve.

Continuing in Mark, we find out what happens when the woman's desperate faith pushes her to seek God's care through Christ.

> When she heard about Jesus, she came up behind him
> in the crowd and touched his cloak,
> because she thought,
> "If I just touch his clothes, I will be healed."
> Immediately her bleeding stopped
> and she felt in her body
> that she was freed from her suffering.
>
> MARK 5:27–29, NIV

After over a decade of prolonged agony and strain, it took only one outstretched hand to end her affliction.

After the woman pours out the contents of her heart, she is trembling at the feet of Christ.

> He said to her, "Daughter, your faith has healed you. Go in peace and be freed from your suffering."
>
> MARK 5:34, NIV

This Scripture reaffirms not only the woman's strong and resilient faith but also the believer's responsibility to seek God out in the crowd. It took seven years of intense internal turmoil for me to realize that I'd lost sight of His presence in my life.

Although physical bleeding was not my complaint, I did bleed from the inside out in another way. Fear and despair left deep-set stains on my psyche and behavior. Just like the unclean woman, some tainted part of me accepted the lie that I was an unsolvable problem to be hidden or cast away. I, too, allowed myself to be called "untouchable" and "incurable." That was until Jesus walked by and changed everything.

This is the story of how God was faithfully moving through every detail of my struggle with and recovery from bipolar disorder type II.

It's a true narrative full of mess, conflict, and confusion. It is not a set of uplifting devotionals or inspiring tales, but a collection of memoirs written in chronological order. There is a beginning, a middle, and an end that you won't want to miss. It is a raw retelling of the trials I faced in the realm of mental illness.

While the struggle itself is a focus, a more important focus is the overcoming of those struggles through faith. Keep these important points in mind:

- See yourself in the toil and strife, but learn from my mistakes!
- Darkness is often unavoidable, but don't lose yourself in it!
- Trouble and misfortune will follow you, but keep your eyes forward!

True faith means to walk with God. As He walked with Adam and Eve in the Garden of Eden, He made a way through His precious Son to walk with you. He wants to hold your hand through it all.

While these contents are meant to be helpful to you, this is *not* a self-help book. Help comes from Him. You might require instruction and correction. Perhaps you wish for healing and redemption. Maybe you long for hope and peace. It's possible that you don't even know, and if you don't, then neither do I. But your Heavenly Father knows. Focus on strengthening your personal relationship with Father, Son, and Spirit; the rest will come in time.

The tried-and-true methods to grow closer to God are Bible study, prayer, and fellowship with other believers. These practices will shed further light on Christ's sacrifice, which should be the foundation of your faith. At the foot of the cross is where you will find what you've been looking for. If I successfully lead you anywhere through the pages of this book, I pray that it is there. No spiritual leader is worth following unless they are first a follower of Christ.

At the end of each chapter, there is a small section reserved for your personal correction and reflection. Read these questions carefully and answer them intentionally. This is your opportunity to choose life. To the readers of this book, here is a prayer for you:

- May you be so comforted by the presence of the Lord that your sin becomes uncomfortable.
- May you be so vulnerable in the presence of the Lord that your greatest weaknesses become His greatest strengths.
- May you come to know Him and love Him more fully, as He knows and loves you.

FOREWORD

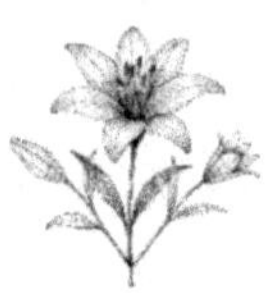

I grew up in the sixties and seventies. In my lifetime, the treatment and societal views of mental health issues have traveled the full spectrum. We have gone from the taboo requiring these few "unfortunates" to hide behind closed doors and "let's not talk about it," to congressional inquiries on the best ways to approach and help our sons and daughters.

Elizabeth is one such current-day success story. She isn't a Hollywood star, professional athlete, or recognized personality. She has stood on the edge, like millions of young Christian Americans, as evil tried with every fiery breath to crush the joy of her victory in Christ. She has battled demons from early childhood to adulthood. She put her trust in God, family, friends, and medical professionals to carry her to where she is today. She is a Christian wife and mother, and my daughter.

Beth and I, as Christian parents, never imagined that one of our children would battle mental health issues, much less write a book about it. My biggest concern as a dad with eight kids was adequately clothing and feeding them to sustain life. The needs of eight kids were voracious, paycheck to paycheck, and anything that wasn't a necessity took a back seat. I would transfer an agreed-upon sum to Beth, and she always managed to provide for household expenses, school activities, and sports. I thank the Lord every day for her parenting and budgeting. She gave the kids a sense of "normalcy". Our kids shared family and household responsibilities, allowing Beth to return to college. She completed a BSN (Bachelor of Science Nursing), MSN (Master of Science in Nursing), FNP (Family Nurse Practitioner), and, more recently, her PMHNP (Psychiatric Mental Health Nurse Practitioner) degree.

I always worried the odds were against us with so many kids. We have been blessed that the children survived relatively unscathed through the gauntlet of childhood disease. It was not unusual for a child to die 100 years ago. Elizabeth is our youngest child, and to be blunt, at the bottom of the food chain. A casual familiarity with the culture of larger families and their exponential interactions, relationships, emotions, behaviors, and conflicts would help one understand the familial weight these children carry daily. It does not have to be sinister or malicious.

The sibling snowball always rolled downhill, searching for the shy, timid, unsure child who seemed to battle every day to hurdle obstacles to her personal and emotional development. It was unstoppable and impactful! Something as simple as asking Elizabeth to walk across a fast-food restaurant to get a package of ketchup was worthy of a Medal of Honor, because in her mind, it represented a waltz with death. Her testimony not only represents hope for the emotionally struggling but a miracle, reflecting a journey guided by a loving God that used her personal circumstances to shape her not only into a wife and mother, but a confident, bold, Christian actively involved in her church and community.

Beth and I had two primary goals for all our children. First and foremost, we wanted each child to receive Salvation by grace through faith (Ephesians 2:8). We wanted their eternal residence to be settled! Second, we aimed to equip them with a Christian backpack full of tools to honor God in their Christian walk and "fight the good fight" (1 Timothy 6:12). We are grateful Elizabeth drew on these tools to keep moving forward.

Regardless of the circumstances, it was up to Elizabeth to make the right choices. She was unique in being the youngest, but her brothers and sisters never held a sibling meeting and voted unanimously to give her a break or take it easy on her. Each one had a stronger, more vocal personality and certainly did not hold back for her benefit.

Elizabeth had to battle to survive. Despite that, in writing this book, she never plays the blame game. It is not a book of excuses. It is a book with true experiences that can provide common ground and hope for millions struggling with mental health and the despair that so often accompanies it.

—Jerry, Author's Father

PART ONE:

The Darkness

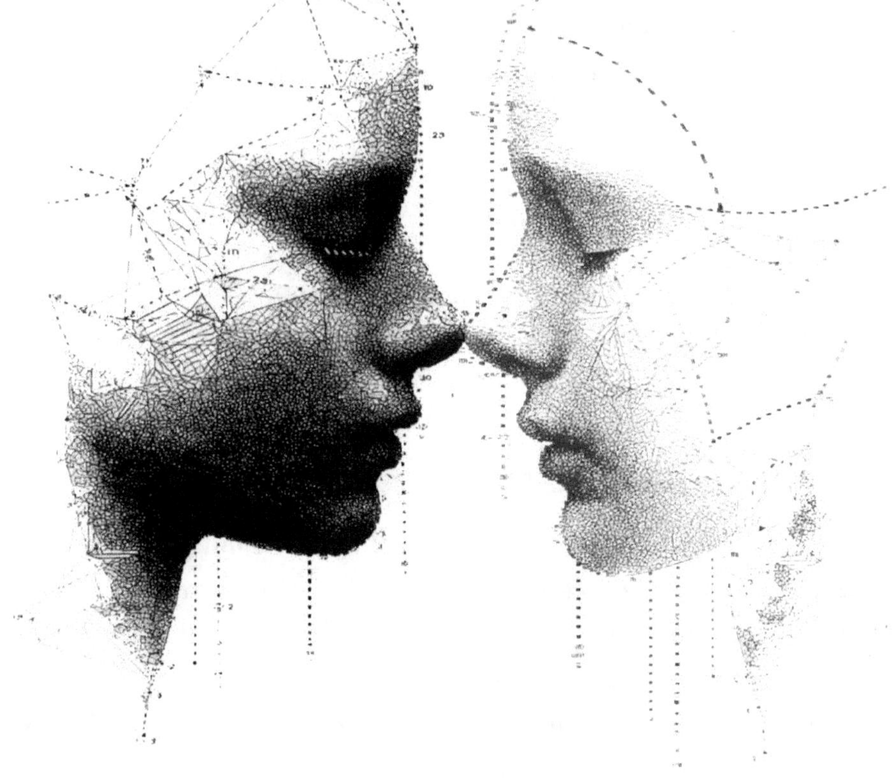

CHAPTER 1

Fear is a Liar

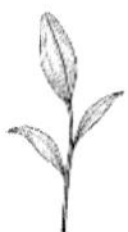

Many of my childhood memories have been tainted by anxiety and fear. Experiences that should have been pleasant and joyous took place in quite the opposite fashion and attitude. Constant uneasiness and nagging apprehension saturated my little soul wherever it traveled. While my school, town, and church environments could have easily nurtured the innocent wonder of childhood, I chose rather to focus on the terrifying what-ifs. Unlike a typical child, I was not blissfully unaware of the dangerous possibilities that swirled all around. In fact, I became increasingly cognizant of the evil in the world and even the evil within me.

AN UNHAPPY TEMPERAMENT

Outside the shelter and safety of home, the risk of harm felt endless. One step off the porch could expose me to a nefarious watching eye. An unwise interaction with someone of bad influence could lead to a mountain of trouble. Simply walking to the park could end in a kidnapping! Although extreme and sensational, these fears plagued me. A spy was never revealed, a peer never led me astray, nor was I ever abducted. Still, I indulged in this irrational fear of injury. It wasn't because I was certain this impending sense of doom would come to pass, but because there was no guarantee it wouldn't. On the off chance an incident of great consequence did occur, I must be prepared to process it appropriately.

In response to this chaotic energy that never seemed to settle, I convinced myself that determined worry could help in mitigating any potential disaster. These threatening characters could be anyone and culminate anywhere, so I was always on guard. It was an attempt to ease the inner turmoil; however, it only intensified it. I could not afford to miss any strangers lurking, monsters hiding, or demons slinking. There had been no adverse or traumatic event to warrant such a magnitude of fear, but my imagination was so vivid that no such event was necessary. Bad things happen to good people all the time; they certainly could happen to me.

This consistent practice of fearing the unknown established a destructive pattern of thought I began to rely on as a sort of superstition. I did not yet know that superstitions hold no merit and their "success" rates are wildly unpredictable. Instead of my worry working as intended—to prevent bad things from happening—it only prepared me for the worst in each new situation. It cultivated a pessimistic attitude and taught me to seek comfort in fear rather than in faith. When things turned out fine, I credited my effort to control rather than crediting God's sovereignty. I lacked the faith to understand that if God *is* in control, there can be nothing to fear.

SPIRITUAL POWERS AND PRINCIPALITIES

The only valid aspect of this pseudo-coping mechanism is the acknowledgment of the supernatural realm and its influence. These forces of evil I feared are quite real and do pose a threat, whether or not this is a widely held belief. Although we cannot see them as we see ourselves, they linger still, perched on the shoulders of adults and children alike.

They prowl outside our homes and along our streets, flying through our cities, intent on deception, perversion, and destruction. They convince non-believers not only that the loving God who created everything doesn't exist, but that they themselves, doing the convincing, don't exist either.

They twist God's perfect design from something that glorifies Him and all that is pure to something that glorifies corruption and separation from Him. They seek tirelessly to disturb peace wherever they can, to distract sinners from their sins, and to do evil for evil's sake.

Paul describes this pressing reality in Ephesians:

> For our struggle is not against flesh and blood, but against the rulers, against the authorities, against the powers of this dark world and against the spiritual forces of evil in the heavenly realms.
>
> EPHESIANS 6:12, NIV

For a God-fearing adult, this is serious business worth thought and consideration. For a child, it can easily feel like life or death. And for me, it did indeed.

Unwarranted and irrational thoughts of abandonment, condemnation, and humiliation tormented me daily. Any legitimate promise of safety was overshadowed by an extreme expectation of harm. This constant provocation ensured my survival instinct was triggered much more than normal. Fighting was not an option for someone as small and powerless as I believed myself to be. There was only the choice to flee from desperate dread or freeze in overwhelming terror. Any extended amount of time spent far from home or family brought on a silent but paralyzing panic. Playdates and sleepovers were usually a catastrophe, ending prematurely with a tearful request to leave. If only I could have conjured the sense to call on the name of Jesus! Unfortunately, such a disordered mind prevented this.

HOW INHERENT SIN GROWS

I spent each day maintaining an unusually delicate balance of sanity. If I wasn't comfortable, then my safety was not assured. When my safety felt uncertain, then panic would rise and threaten to make everything worse. Elementary school was no exception to this rule—in fact, the social and academic demands only added to my discomfort. It was simple enough to follow instructions from a teacher, but the words and actions of my peers were much less predictable. To avoid conflict and ridicule, I kept mostly to myself. Isolation made it easier to manage the raging battle inside.

However, it grew increasingly more difficult to get a handle on these overwhelming emotions. The flurry of early childhood activity was like a stereo at full volume that no amount of freezing could quiet. It forced me to find other ways to cope, or, rather, to run away. Trying to escape this looming cloud of anxiety, I became an impulsive and frantic liar. Any excuse to abandon ship before the school day was over was utilized emphatically. A slight pain during recess turned into a twisted ankle that required medical attention. Butterflies fluttering in my tummy became the start of a contagious stomach flu.

I could have been awarded an Oscar for my many, very convincing performances in pursuit of avoiding anything and anyone that made me uncomfortable! Through this endeavor to soothe the pulsing angst in my heart, I learned how to dramatize, exaggerate, and lie effectively. The most believable excuses were those with as much plausibility as possible. Anything that occurred out of the ordinary, I used to my advantage and detriment. And so, you see how easily fear, unchecked, turns into the ugly, rearing head of sin. The book of James describes how inherent sin is fed by the evil desire in our hearts and then watered by our choices.

> Then, after desire has conceived, it gives birth to sin;
> and sin, when it is full-grown, gives birth to death.
> JAMES 1:15, NIV

To explore care or express concern for something is not automatically wrong. However, letting care and concern morph into powerful fear and anxiety, which can blur the lines of morality, is wrong.

My particular temperament made it especially challenging to exist optimistically and resiliently. It bred a selfish desire to preserve my own comfort and ease above all else. Ironically, there was no care or concern for how my actions might have affected those around me. Instead of resisting the temptation to manipulate others, I did whatever it took to get my way. It's sad but true: Although children are viewed as innocent, they are not without sin. They must be taught the difference between right and wrong, and they must be corrected when they inevitably choose wrong.

The anxiety-fueled behaviors I continually indulged in, refusing to extend the boundaries of my comfort zone, were harming myself and others around me. So, they eventually warranted corrective action. My mother was probably tired of explaining away my lack of social interest and developmentally inappropriate attachment to her. My father was probably irritated by calls from school and "sick days" interrupting his much-needed sleep as a third-shift worker. It's possible they were also increasingly worried about my internal well-being and my ability to function normally, not only in the present but also in the future. If I failed to walk in victory through simple childhood conflict, how could I walk in victory through more complicated contests as an adult?

ORDER AND PERSPECTIVE

Unsurprisingly, my father and I had multiple conversations pertaining to my troublesome behavior. He was not usually an openly tender individual, so when he offered heartfelt advice, it was a serious opportunity. These personal revelations from him went a long way in helping me help myself. I thought of these conversations and interactions whenever the urge to give in to my old ways resurfaced.

On one such instance, while I expressed a dreadful reluctance to return to school after a bout of (genuine) illness, he was inquisitive. "Elizabeth, why do you want to hang around this boring house all day?" he jested.

I sat down on the kitchen floor next to him after he instructed me to do so. The only answer I could muster was, "I don't think this house is boring."

He chuckled a little and replied sharply, "Boring or not, you're supposed to be at school." His response made my mouth go dry as he revealed my staycation would end soon. Then his gaze and body language softened, and he said, "I'd rather not go to work every day, but I have to. Everybody has to do things they don't want to do. It’s what makes the world go 'round."

Despite my immaturity, I understood what he meant and how it applied to my situation. Our family depended on Dad's work to make ends meet. Without it, we would become homeless and starve. If everyone stopped working simply because they disliked it, life would descend into absolute chaos. I pictured overflowing garbage cans and empty grocery store shelves. My father's dedication as a provider was inspirational and encouraging to me, even if it was not a role particularly relatable to me. No one was relying on me to pay the bills, but I had been given an important role to fulfill, too. It was my duty to push through and overcome, like so many had done before me. Emotions, however overwhelming, did not negate my responsibility.

On another occasion, during one of those infamous phone calls home from school, he was uncharacteristically empathetic.

"Sweetie, I used to call my mom from school all the time after my dad died!" he exclaimed.

I'd heard the story of my grandfather, who passed from cancer when my father was only eleven, so I knew he wasn't feigning understanding to placate my distress. It helped the hurt along, realizing I had something in common with the strongest man I knew. As tears ran fast down my cheeks, he continued.

"You can call me whenever you're sad or afraid, as long as you promise to stay at school. Just remember, Mom and I will always be here. We're not going anywhere."

My father's experience of losing a parent, a truly devastating event, made me believe I could push myself harder to manage seven hours of school each day.

FREEDOM AND POTENTIAL

While Dad was wisdom and discipline, Mom was comfort and adventure. Being the youngest of eight children, it was her last opportunity to be "Mom," the one you turn to when you want to laugh or need to cry. She made me feel safe in an unsafe world. During fits of laughter, she was my best friend. Reflecting on her words of wisdom, she was my greatest mentor. The distinction between these roles was clear and exactly what I needed. She recognized when it was time for reassurance and when it was time for some independence. Certainly, her experience raising seven siblings before me proved useful.

She possessed a passion and a calling for the musical arts that took her back to college. Around the time she re-enrolled, I started first grade. Conveniently, when I couldn't summon the courage to attend my school, Mom let me tag along with her instead. It was more manageable to explore new and unfamiliar places outside our home with someone I trusted. Some might see it as coddling or enabling, but truthfully, it was incredibly freeing for me to hold her hand a little while longer. Our bond only strengthened as we spent more time together. Being encompassed by the majesty and harmony of classical music alongside my favorite person was a kind of therapy.

My mother assisted me in any way she could, but she shared one particularly memorable strategy with me. It was simple, yet incredibly effective at chasing away fear. Consistent with her love for music, she suggested I fight my battles with a song. It went like this:

When I am afraid, I will trust in you, trust in you.
When I am afraid, I will trust in you
'cause Jesus is my God.

I didn't expect something so silly and childish to do much. However, as I walked to a friend's house one day, the hum of distress set in, and there was only this song to hold on to. Even silently singing in my head caused the buzzing to subside and the fear to melt away as if it never existed. This small act of faith brought me peace, hope, and even excitement!

The reason these words were so powerful in the face of fear was because of their holy origin. Unbeknownst to me, these verses I recited could be found in the book of Psalms:

When I am afraid, I put my trust in you.
In God, whose word I praise—
[cont'd next page]

in God I trust and am not afraid.
What can mere mortals do to me?
PSALM 56:3–4, NIV

I must have customized the last line in my version, as it is obviously not present in the original Psalm, but it still worked out. I was essentially declaring the name of Jesus over my situation and adopting that authority enabled me to be brave.

It was clear how fiercely my mother loved me. I tried my best to cherish the closeness in our relationship because it was unique and special. Neither my siblings nor my peers were allowed the opportunity to spend so much quality time with such a beloved parent. The surplus of attention they paid me may lead some to believe I was over-indulged, but spoiled children aren't thankful, and attention and love go hand in hand. I was deeply grateful for her loving acceptance of me.

She thoughtfully adapted to the eccentricity that accompanied my extreme introversion. An affectionate mother is one of the cornerstones of a happy and healthy childhood. It pains me to think of how much more I could have suffered if not for the light of my mother's unconditional love.

SUPPORTING NEW GIFTS AND MAKING HEADWAY

Another light that gleamed in my life came from an affinity for the creative. Literature, cinema, music, and visual art were exceedingly attractive. I took to reading like a fish to water, devouring books often late into the night. Movies brought those stories to life in such an intentional way that they quickly mesmerized me.

Although I shared my mother's adoration for music and played a few different instruments sporadically, visual art was my primary interest and particular gift. I tried my hand at any and every medium with great purpose and pleasure. Artistic expressions became an avenue to tranquility that helped me better process and connect to my surroundings.

Through a pen, pencil, or paintbrush, I could translate my chaotic introspection into something that made sense. Because of the sheer volume of my thoughts, countless roads in my mind had gone untraveled. These untraveled roads bothered me terribly, but the physical exertion of my hands creating images on paper or canvas somehow quieted that constant preoccupation. Steep mountains towering over a lush valley with a winding stream not only portrayed a beautiful natural landscape but also a plane of peace in me. Less organized and structured, but equally compelling, black and white abstract scribbles surrounding a lone shadowy figure conveyed how lost I sometimes felt. Whether good or bad, beautiful or ugly, understood or misunderstood, every piece came from the heart and was precious to me.

Whenever I escaped the classroom, you could find me in the corner with art supplies to occupy my soul. I enjoyed every second. It lessened my burden of fear. However, despite my wishes, it wasn't possible to skip school and play make-believe every day. Slowly, with age, experience, and compassionate parents, my confidence in the familiar and mildly unfamiliar grew. Although I still occasionally tapped out of disagreeable situations, my parents' aid and accommodation during this stage of life were lasting. Their example of faith, along with my gift of creativity, carried me through more difficult times to come.

PROS AND CONS OF A LARGE FAMILY

Yes, there were difficult times. Even happy children in healthy homes experience challenges. I was not always happy, and our home could have been healthier, so of course, we faced hardship. There were financial concerns, circumstantial instability, and spiritual battles. My father solely supported his larger-than-average family at a job he sorely disliked. There was always provision, but rarely excess, so my siblings and I had a paper route to fund most extracurricular activities. My mother did not enjoy living in the Midwest, which was far from her extended family, and the long, harsh winters were an intense adjustment. Even though we stayed put for thirteen years, there was always talk of moving here or there. Both parents had to lean hard on the Lord through seasons of loss, illness, and moral dilemma.

Raising eight children must have been overwhelming. As a sibling, it was sometimes crushing to grow up in such a full house. Seven distinct personalities and temperaments to be mindful of throughout the day; seven sets of preferences and opinions to remember for fear of insulting or offending. My parents were being pulled in seven or more directions, which often left little room for me to vie with the demands of others. My dad used to say, "It's always something." I'd say basic statistics would confirm that theory. Often, I felt like just another face in our crowded family.

None of this scarred or traumatized me by any means. Surely, it bred resilience. But it also bred jealousy, antipathy, and bitterness between us siblings. These unspoken feelings cultivated a climate of unhealthy competition. Win at all costs. My brothers physically fought in anger daily. My sisters argued and put each other down often. Even though they were scolded or punished, it stopped only briefly. I learned it was the way of our family to bite or get bitten. Cornered animals are expected to defend themselves. So, I engaged in this behavior too, even though it made me feel rotten.

Eventually, my defensive efforts transformed into offensive attacks after being cornered one too many times. It is said that hurt people hurt people, and this couldn't have been truer of my character in our family. Unfortunately, this ugly practice overflowed into relationships outside the home, resulting in the insensitive treatment of others because I lacked the courage to be different. We might have seen ourselves as "tough," but a more accurate description would be "downright mean." Instead of finding strength in humility by the examples set before me, I found strength in pride.

It's unclear if there was anything practical my parents could have done to prevent or stop this attitude. Freedom from the chains of sin and failure is not found in blame. Yes, there was room for improvement, but they tried and ultimately succeeded in providing a safe place for us to grow up.

My parents' flaws and shortcomings only pointed to their need for a savior, just like me. Aside from the questionable practices and behaviors my siblings and I engaged in, we were good kids. Our goodness obviously didn't come from within but from the God who surrounded us in His grace and forgiveness.

Progressives might say, "Have fewer children." Still, being the youngest in a large family, I cannot even theoretically agree with that opinion. Families can be happy or unhappy, unrelated to their size.

It would be impossible for parents to know how far they could be stretched if they did not stretch at all. My parents have earned commendations for their generosity in having and raising us, not scrutiny. Even though it was difficult, I wouldn't go back and change it, especially not by hypothetically subtracting one of my siblings from existence.

The birth of eight souls is also, potentially, the rebirth of eight souls through Christ, furthering the reach of the Kingdom of God to redeem and reunite. As He declares in the book of Jeremiah:

> "For I know the plans I have for you," declares the LORD,
> "plans to prosper you and not to harm you,
> plans to give you hope and a future."
> JEREMIAH 29:11, NIV

Who are you or I, merely created beings, to question or contemplate the Creator's divine intention for the people He has given life to?

Aside from all the relational discord and personality clashes, there were many enjoyable times in my family, too! We made wonderful memories wherever we went. When we laughed, we laughed until we cried, and our bellies ached. When we played, we played by the rules, and it was fair. At the dinner table each evening, we shared pieces of ourselves that restored the balance between the danger of the world and the safety of our home.

We always found a way back to family unity, no matter who messed up, what they did, or how grumpy it made our father. We made allowances for each other's faults and chose to love and be loyal, above all else. And again, it wasn't through our own righteousness or integrity that this was accomplished, but because we were taught biblical standards of truth.

A FIRM FOUNDATION

The foundation of a child's fortitude is laid by their familial environment. Innocent babies, born into a world of darkness, grow to reflect the quality of their childhoods and the faithful or unfaithful guardians charged with protecting them. One's childhood experience can be perceived as generally good or bad, but the spectrum between those two is wide.

God knows and sees everything, big and small. Even for someone whose foundation of fortitude was laid cracked, unstable, or rotten, there is good news. That foundation can be re-laid and renewed, independent of the past, by faith in God, guaranteed with eternal life through Jesus Christ.

It is enlightening to know that, despite my family's many imperfections, it was a blessing to be placed with them. I used to wish for parents with more time or more money, but hindsight is 20/20. I realize now that my parents' spiritual direction, living in a Christ-centered home, was worth far more than any fleeting desire or foolish comparison in my heart. I was given an advantage in life that many children are not. My parents set their sights on Heaven rather than on the world. They gave me the tools to discover that God can turn any failure, big or small, into overwhelming success.

Start children off on the way they should go,
and even when they are old they will not turn from it.
PROVERBS 22:6, NIV

REFLECTION AND CORRECTION

Fear is a Liar

List three fears, past or present, that have shaken or weakened your faith.

Have any fear-based decisions resulted from your lack of faith? What were the outcomes of those decisions? How did they push you further from God's presence?

Declare how God delivered you, or will deliver you, from these fears.

____

____

____

____

____

____

In the following verses, where an emphasis has been added, discover the tools given to help us in overcoming fear.

Do not be anxious about anything, but in every situation,
by **prayer and petition**, with thanksgiving,
present your requests to God . . .
PHILIPPIANS 4:6, NIV [EMPHASIS ADDED]

Have I not commanded you? Be strong and courageous.
Do not be afraid; do not be discouraged,
for the Lord your God **will be with you wherever you go.**
JOSHUA 1:9, NIV [EMPHASIS ADDED]

Peace I leave with you; my peace I give you.
I do not give to you as the world gives.
Do not let your hearts be troubled and do not be afraid.
JOHN 14:27, NIV [EMPHASIS ADDED]

DO NOT BE	HE GIVES US
Anxious	P ________________ and P ________________
Discouraged	P ________________
Troubled or afraid	P ________________

Meditate on this next passage of scripture by reading it silently, reciting it aloud, and finally writing it down:

> For God has not given us a spirit of fear,
> but of power and of love and of a sound mind.
> 2 TIMOTHY 1:7, NKJV

In prayer, ask God to search your heart for any fear that offends Him. Journal what you receive below:

God tells us not to fear 365 times in the Bible. That's how many days there are in a year! It's as if He's urging us to live without fear each and every day.

Regardless of interpretation, we can be certain that fear does not come from God, who is perfect and good. Fear comes from our imperfect and sinful nature. Sometimes the enemy can manipulate situations or perpetuate thoughts that encourage fear, but God gives us His Spirit of power, love, and a sound mind to choose faith every time.

CHAPTER 2

God is Good All the Time

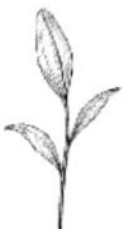

Around the age of twelve, things really started changing. Interestingly, I both do and don't mean the cliché transformation of puberty. Yes, adolescence is a difficult, awkward, and uncomfortable time in human life. My puberty was physically, mentally, and emotionally typical. However, this other change was much more abstract and undefined. There was a spiritual shift I did not understand, or even initially recognize in the slightest. Something big was coming that had the potential to drive me further down a path of darkness.

DIVINE DEVELOPMENT

I had first prayed for salvation six years prior and did, indeed, receive God's gift of eternal life that day. After a brief conversation with my mother, I knelt at my bedside, head bowed, and eyes closed. The prayer began with a declaration of what I believed to be true of God: He sent His only son, Jesus, to die on the cross for my sins, and He rose again on the third day. I asked Him, "Please forgive me of all my sins," understanding His authority to accomplish that fully. Finally, I welcomed Him into my heart and asked Him to guide me for the rest of my life.

As I sat on the carpet, the late afternoon sunlight streamed through the window and shone on my skin. It seemed to warm me from the inside out like never before. It was a tangible hug from an invisible being, the Holy Spirit. He enveloped and sealed me in His presence, self-existent and all-redemptive, as He does for all those He saves—for God is perfect light and perfect love. Praying "Amen" and opening my eyes, I remember thinking, *That's it? That's all I have to do? Why doesn't everyone do this?* Oh, the innocence and purity of childhood faith!

Regardless of when and where it is received, salvation is truly so simple and easy to accept. A passage in Romans describes how we can receive this gift:

> If you declare with your mouth, "Jesus is Lord,"
> and believe in your heart that God raised him
> from the dead, you will be saved.
> For it is with your heart that you believe and are justified,
> and it is with your mouth that you profess your faith
> and are saved.
>
> ROMANS 10:9–10, NIV

My six-year-old musings were not mistaken, despite how much they might be overshadowed later in my life.

Young Elizabeth hadn't yet encountered the hardship that her twelve-year-old self was becoming well acquainted with. Apart from typical adolescent adjustments, there were also circumstantial changes that would begin to affect me greatly. The sudden transition from childhood faith to ceaseless doubt was spurred on by deep sadness and profound unhappiness. Anxiety was also involved—in fact, we had become inseparable friends. Fear was how the devil got a foothold in my life, but despair was how he held me captive for many years to come, eternally saved or not.

DISEASE AND DOUBT

The onslaught of these more intense feelings coincided with the diagnosis of my father's illness, scleroderma. Scleroderma is an incredibly rare autoimmune disease that causes the immune system to attack its own tissues. While "tissues" commonly refers to the layers of the skin, the term can also include blood vessels, muscles, bones, and internal organs. Unfortunately for my father, his case presented aggressively, progressively, and all-inclusively. The doctor who offered this diagnosis gave him five years to live.

Understandably, this came as a tremendous shock to the entire family, myself included. The man hardly caught a cold or got the flu, let alone a mystery disorder with a death sentence. It broke my heart to see him in physical pain and inner turmoil. It discouraged me to see his health visually deteriorate. His skin started tightening up and stretching taut, especially around jointed areas, as if he'd been injected with Botox all over. But, unlike the popular anti-aging beauty treatment, the condition put him through extreme daily pain and took away much of his ability to function normally.

The world turned upside down, and the one absolute I had relied on most, my father's strength, seemed to slip away. Change is difficult in almost every capacity, especially when change comes in the form of loss (if not a loss of life, then at least a loss of quality of life). It was the loss of stability that led to this even deeper level of insecurity in me. Pessimism struck again! I asked myself, "If the strongest of the strong could be cut down in an instant, how can the weak ever survive?"

A newfound awareness of the fragility of life shattered any confidence I'd previously gained. Typically, I would've leaned on my parents' resilience to remain steady, but this time, they were just as shaken. Their struggle to accept their permanently changed reality was painfully obvious. However, they quickly toughened up and got on with whatever adaptations were necessary to continue. Instead of moving along with them, I found myself stuck and desperately grasping for reasons why.

Even if these concerns were vocalized, I likely wouldn't have accepted any of the answers to ease my dismay. Sorrow was welcomed into my heart through a wide-open door. Old wounds oozed bitterness and offense, which led me to believe somehow my father's diagnosis was justified. I entertained the lie that perhaps his pain and suffering were punishment for his shortcomings. In my mind, God's lack of intervention illustrated His lack of care for my family and me.

Thus, the dominoes began to fall. My body and mind were advancing too rapidly for me to comprehend. My father was struck with a severe illness. Nobody told me what would or wouldn't happen.

As if on the wind, questions and doubts appeared around the goodness of God I had previously and confidently regarded as true. In a divine, tailored counterargument to this inner tension, we find in Matthew:

> "Lord, if it's you," Peter replied,
> "tell me to come to you on the water."
> "Come," he said. Then Peter got down out of the boat,
> walked on the water and came toward Jesus.
> But when he saw the wind, he was afraid
> and, beginning to sink, cried out, "Lord, save me!"
> Immediately Jesus reached out his hand and caught him.
> "You of little faith," he said, "why did you doubt?"
> MATTHEW 14:28–31, NIV

Like Peter walking on the water with Jesus, my eyes looked everywhere but ahead at Him, my Lord and Savior, and I started drowning in a sea of doubt.

DESPAIR AND DEPRESSION

It was as if someone had turned out the lights in slow motion. The darkness didn't come quickly: it was terribly, terribly slow. It fell upon me like a candle left to burn out on its own. So slowly, I struggled to remember the characteristics and aspects of previously enjoyable and beloved light.

Love? What was love? Light? Where was it? Everything became dull and drab. Even colors lost their saturation. The pencils and paints that used to bring me such clarity now lie flat, jumbled, and lifeless on the paper.

Life that year was a blur. I went to school, returned home, and went to sleep. There weren't even tears, just a quiet, gray, and meaningless existence. It was like my body went on living, leaving my soul behind. With no motivation or purpose, I moved on autopilot and fulfilled obligations to the bare minimum. Homework and chores were completed carelessly compared to my previous passion and prudence. The amount of energy invested in a task no longer mattered; my goal was simply to keep going. So, I droned on, day after day, season after season.

Anyone familiar with the signs and symptoms of depression could recognize my ailment easily. Persistent sadness and hopelessness, loss of interest and motivation, and excessive anxiety and irritability were present in me for all to see, even if they weren't visible to me. Certainly, there was a noticeable deficiency, but there was no need to name or identify the problem yet.

I thought I was a victim of unfortunate circumstances, and whenever those circumstances changed for the better, I would too. My dad was sick and dying. If he were healed, everything would go back to normal, and the darkness would retreat.

However, with complex and chronic diseases, a swift recovery is as rare as the disease itself, if it even happens at all. My parents sought the best care available, often driving over eleven hours to consult with specialists. Despite my father receiving proper medical treatment, all they could do was slow down the disease's progression. The goal was to minimize damage by prolonging the disorder from reaching vital tissues and life-sustaining organs. Nothing could reverse any previous harm or prevent further harm from occurring. In short, treatment would only buy him more time.

Despite the overwhelming nature of this crisis, circumstances improved slowly but surely. Medications kicked in while physical therapy provided my father relief. As financial provision came through, his five-year prognosis started to extend conservatively. My family could breathe again, no longer afraid that we could lose our father at any moment. Outcomes became even more promising when talks about moving to a warmer climate were seriously entertained. But this intervention was unexpected and unwelcome from my point of view. I wanted things to go back to normal, not forward into a new normal.

It was plainly understandable that this disease would kill Dad eventually, and nothing could be done to stop it. The helplessness and hopelessness that came with facing such a definite bottom line were vast. My state of mind continued to worsen as I slipped deeper into the hole of depression. Spirits of misery and grief blinded me from seeing the blessings amidst this hardship. God's mercies were clearly plentiful, but I couldn't get past my misguided belief that He had unfairly shortened my father's life. Ultimately, my father's fate lay solely in God's hands, whom I had begun to distrust emphatically.

Once the darkness was permitted to exert its power over me, the mental and emotional disturbances transformed from mostly uncomfortable to almost unbearable. I experienced the worsening effects in these ways:

- Anxiety morphed into panic.
- The slightest conflict became the end of the world.
- Wallowing was not enough, and I soon turned to sobbing uncontrollably.
- Crying-induced migraines became a regular occurrence.
- Antisocial tendencies graduated to a level of complete reclusiveness.
- Family and friends started calling me "hermit."
- Idleness consumed me, and I stared at nothing, paralyzed, for hours.

Even the concept of time was distorted into something insignificant and unimportant. The sooner the days were over, the better. Sleep was a dream, and waking up was a nightmare. My roots in reality were rotting.

DISCOVERY OF DARKNESS

Sometime in my thirteenth year, I started reconsidering the assumption that my experience was typical and temporary. It felt too intense, too debilitating, and too prolonged. I questioned:

- Why do activities that once brought satisfaction and glee now only reflect the numbness inside?
- Why can't I relate to my peers anymore, or happily take part in their careless fun and games?

- Why haven't I grown out of the suspicion that something is seriously wrong with me?

It was all so disorienting, but something deep inside—too hushed and far away to be called a voice, however similar—prompted me to seek answers.

So, I did what most kids did in 2013 as pioneer consumers of the internet age—I googled it. In the privacy of my bedroom, a quest for answers commenced. The results of the Google search, probably along the lines of "Why am I so sad all the time?" were surprisingly straightforward. The word "depression" was consistently present in all the links and articles. It felt like a light bulb lit up above my head. Something clicked, and quickly the dots connected. I remember thinking, "Why didn't I see this before?" My troubled spirit had a name, Depression, and now I could figure out what it wanted from me.

My mother had just recently uncovered the origin of her own occasional suffering to be seasonal depression. This added another piece to the puzzle. My mother's forthcomingness in sharing her experience introduced me to the idea of the "little happy pill" she took in the winter, which helped her tremendously. Part of me indulged in wondering, only for a moment, if that could be a solution for me, too. However, another Google search and a documentary on medicated children quickly put me off the idea. I didn't desire to be changed; I simply wanted a reprieve.

I may have stewed on this information for a bit of time, holding onto hope the depression would go away on its own. Vulnerable conversations were one thing I endeavored to avoid as long as possible. Walls had already been constructed around my opinions and feelings. Somewhere between scleroderma and my preceding pre-teen years, Mom and Dad ceased to be my heroes. Part of me wished they would come to the rescue, but a bigger part argued I could rescue myself. Ultimately, I conceded to sound judgment and sought help despite my discomfort. Considering my worsening predicament, perhaps this only postponed the inevitable.

DISAPPOINTMENT AND DETERMINATION

Reluctantly and impulsively, I sought my mother one evening, an emotional mess. Through tears, I confessed to the unexplained sadness and hopelessness I'd been feeling and not knowing what to do about it.

- I *yearned* for comfort from her through kind words or a loving hug.
- I *hoped* she would want to know more and ask questions.
- I *craved* interest and attention from her, reminiscent of the past.
- I *wished* she would see me, more so than she had recently.

But she didn't. The mom who had held her daughter's hand through separation anxiety no longer had an available hand to extend in this. I approached knowing her plate was full, but counting on room for just a little bit more. Although there was genuine concern in her eyes when she looked at me, it was resigned. Bruised, battered, and with a sigh of defeat, all she said was, "Do you want to try some medication?"

The rosy, dreamy image I'd conjured up of things going back to the way they were when Mom and I were friends instantly dissipated. Instead, I saw a sterilized version of our relationship as we gave up laboring and found ourselves enslaved to modern medicine. We'd experienced enough of that with Dad! I felt a responsibility to proceed with immense caution, for fear this terrible vision might come true.

Suddenly, the facade of maturity I'd been entertaining became necessary for survival. I dried my tears, pulled myself together, and replied with a weak but firm "No." I quickly found myself climbing back up the stairs I'd only just come down. On the journey down, there was hope for light, but on the defeated journey back up, there was only a return to darkness. Yes, indeed, this burden was mine alone to carry.

This cut-short interaction could have ended more positively. If consideration and sensitivity on behalf of my mother had been included in my plan, perhaps some of her defensive walls might have fallen. Bricks of fear, obligation, and pain hardened my mother's heart. If I had shown an understanding of her struggle, she might have been freer to understand mine. It wasn't difficult to imagine the sorrow of a wife who had lost part of her husband. I knew, even amid my own hurt, she was hurting too.

Desire for comfort, interest, and attention did not apply only to me. The key to healthy relationships is a focus on what can be given, rather than what can be received. When all parties implement this practice, no cup is left empty. My despair and anguish equipped me perfectly to console my mother in her own despair and anguish. If only I had the spiritual insight to be selfless first. Denying the goodness of God denied Him access to my heart. He could perfectly fill my cup with anything I needed, but I never held it out for Him to do so.

DIVISIONAL DIFFERENCES

Aside from depression and a dismal home life, there were also social expectations at school and in the community at large that kept me stumbling. I'd attended the same public school, in the same tiny Iowa town, since first grade. There was only one local K–12 establishment, so most of my peers had been there from the beginning, too. The consistency and familiarity of being with the same sixty students every year were helpful, but sometimes stifling. There was no anonymity to hide behind. Everyone knew everyone because there weren't very many people to know!

In this minuscule city of around 1,800 people, one only needed a surname to recall the corresponding street of residence, place of employment, or general reputation. This kind of intimacy may seem cozy in theory, but for intimacy to be safe, grace and acceptance are required. The lack of these qualities manifested in rumors, backstories, and gossip attached to each family. Everyone seemed to know of some dirt worth digging up, a tragedy worth speaking in hushed tones over, or an unfortunate circumstance that generally marred. My family wasn't exempt from being made the object of this game, even by Christians who knew better.

We were set apart from that place in some uncomfortably obvious ways. It was uncommon to have more than a few kids there, much less eight! Our faithful and devoted aversion to participating in communal activities, like dances, resulted in social isolation. Any allowed participation was restricted. Those restrictions gradually loosened later on, but first impressions are lasting impressions. Many viewed us as weirdly religious, ultra-conservative, and culturally estranged.

My mother and father didn't drink, which was a subject of division in a social setting where adult entertainment was composed largely of sports and alcohol. Fortunately, athletics were an enjoyable and encouraged familial strong suit. Most of us siblings excelled in multiple competitive endeavors, which granted us a great deal of conditional acceptance. If we hadn't had sports, we might have been outcasts. My parents shouldered any unfair speculation as gracefully as they could, but it had to have hurt them, too. Despite developing several loving and understanding relationships, it didn't affect their future decision to move far away.

DISGUISES AND DANCES

My experience in middle school wasn't much better. Early on, I learned that parents who would scold a son or daughter for unkindness often created unkindness in the children themselves. Youth learned much more from modeled behavior and overheard conversations than from lectures. If those parents had understood just how adept their children were at imitating behavior, would they have checked their tongues and attitudes? In my experience, they were unaware or simply apathetic, because generational spirits of judgment and pride leaped into the hearts of the next generation—my generation—in full force.

I was bullied. Not nearly as bad as so many others, but it happened nonetheless. Put-downs, exclusions, poorly timed jokes, and cruel pranks were not uncommon. Shamefully, I was also a bully myself at times. The habits picked up at home from older siblings and the ones I went along with at school certainly earned me the title.

This weed of bullying wasn't a new sprout in the garden of junior high. It had been growing young and pliable roots underground for years. Changing priorities and standards became the fertilizer this ugly plant needed to grow rampant.

A superficial and immature hierarchical system was established in this latest kingdom of schooling. Value was no longer placed on who could run the fastest or ace the spelling test. Achievement was still important, but appearance crowned the queen. There was always a snide comment to be made about someone's clothing, hair, or weight. An overemphasis on materialism and lookism poisoned my and others' ability to define worthiness. Consequently, I harbored significant personal insecurity, much like many others would, and cared a great deal too much about what others thought of me. My estimation of worth depended on all but my relationship with God.

This maintenance became very difficult, since the deep ideological dilemmas confronted in depression were drenched in empty ideals of status. I wanted to shout, "I'm drowning!" but my friends at the time only cared if my swimsuit was name-brand. So, I continued with the guise that everything was okay. Okay, enough, at least, to keep up with the ever-changing trends. Maintaining the façade wasted valuable energy, I realized, which would be much better spent elsewhere.

I was tired, literally and figuratively, of playing the game with others, which included a series of lies.

- The lies I told to fit in:
  "Oh, I've watched that show! It's actually my favorite."
- The lies I told to impress:
  "I met so many new friends on our family vacation."
- The lies I told to deter ridicule:
  "I don't miss my mom. I skipped school to help out with something important. Not that it's any of your business."

These deceptions haunted my thoughts and stared back at me when I looked in the mirror, spiritually convicted. I'd been caught in these lies and endured awkward silence when faced with unanswerable questions one too many times. It forced me to question the purpose of it all.

A lie will always be a lie, no matter how far it's taken or how ardently it's believed. This change in perspective drove me into the arms of loneliness. Nothing I had ever done or said was for anyone but myself.

A few eye-opening experiences, including an intense anti-bullying assembly, featuring a classmate who included my name with the notorious group of mean girls, led me to clean up my act. For my own sake and that of others, I distanced myself from anyone unrepentantly cruel. The process wasn't as conscious and intentional as it sounds, though. Under the secret thumb of depression, what could be construed as a calculated decision from the outside was really a gasp for air on the inside.

Smaller, newer friend groups were formed. Circles within circles, where some of us could find relief from the past and consolation in shared perspectives. It was at this time that I made truly lasting friendships with people who remain close to my heart, simply because we were honest with one another. God had mercy on me, and loneliness loosened its grip. These quality-over-quantity relationships began filling the hole of loss at home.

O DEATH, WHERE IS THY STING?

Fathers are called to be providers and protectors. My father fulfilled that calling until his decline in health forced him to step away from the role. Through the divine work of Providence, my mother was able to replace him as breadwinner. With a medical career she never pictured for herself, Mom's supplemental income became our primary income. Despite my dad's blatant discontentment with disability and early retirement, I actually experienced a kind of relief from this. He had been a sufficient provider, but I witnessed him struggle to find a balance between responsibility and passion. Defeat in that regard often left him stressed out, unpredictably moody, and generally failing to regulate his emotions. Hopefully, with less obligation and more independence, despite enduring pain, he might make whatever time he had left intentional and satisfactory.

Despite our collective lack of acknowledgement, it was a blessing for my father—a non-stop, "always doing something" kind of man—to be challenged with stillness. When face-to-face with the uncontrollable and unchangeable, it would be wiser to focus on what's in store rather than what has already passed. This is where the wondrous, redeeming power of God moves freely.

One day, my father's body will finally fail him, and we will be separated from each other for a time. Whatever grief may overcome me then, 1 Thessalonians says:

> Brothers and sisters, we do not want you to be uninformed about those who sleep in death, so that you do not grieve like the rest of mankind, who have no hope. For we believe that Jesus died and rose again, and so we believe that God will bring with Jesus those who have fallen asleep in him.
>
> 1 THESSALONIANS 4:13–14, NIV

Holding to faith, we believe death is not the end for Christians. Whatever cannot be redeemed in this life shall certainly be redeemed in the next. The same body that once failed my father will be resurrected and made new, free of pain, free of restriction, and free of disease. His spirit, preserved through Jesus Christ, will be reunited with his body made new, and he will meet his family again in wholeness and holiness.

REFLECTION AND CORRECTION

God is Good All the Time

Everyone will experience loss at some point in their life. This hardship is not limited to losing a loved one; loss of employment, standing, home, health, and/or innocence are other examples of loss.

Describe, in heartfelt detail, a personal experience of loss.

There's nothing wrong with feeling sad, angry, or fearful. The problem lies in dwelling in sadness, anger, or fear and letting those emotions lead.

Emotions are God-given. In His life and ministry, Jesus Himself exhibits a wide spectrum of emotion. One of the shortest, yet most powerful, verses in the Bible is:

> Jesus wept.
>
> JOHN 11:35, NIV

Jesus wept for Mary and Martha, who were in anguish over the death of their brother, Lazarus. Unbeknownst to the sisters, Jesus allowed Lazarus to die to exhibit His glory and power, as the Son of God, by raising him from the dead. He knew the sisters would be reunited with their brother and all would be well soon.

Still, being moved by their grief, He wept.

Both Mary and Martha were understandably upset, but their responses to Jesus's late arrival differ slightly. Notice what Martha says that Mary does not.

> When Mary reached the place where Jesus was
> and saw him, she fell at his feet and said,
> "Lord, if you had been here,
> my brother would not have died."
>
> JOHN 11:32, NIV

> "Lord," Martha said to Jesus, "if you had been here,
> my brother would not have died.
> But I know that even now God will give you
> whatever you ask."
>
> JOHN 11:21–22, NIV

This comparison is not to say one sister had greater faith than the other, but this points to an application we can use in our own grief today. Declaring the sovereignty and goodness of God amidst grief is a powerful antidote.

In attempting to grasp an understanding of His sovereignty, we may, at one moment, ask God, "Why did you allow this to happen?" At the very next moment, we must also remember and cling tightly to the undeniable goodness of our God, which transforms our question into a statement: "God, I don't know why you allowed this bad thing to happen, but I believe you will bring goodness and glory out of it, nonetheless."

When we grieve faithfully, loss doesn't pull us away from God but draws us closer.

Identify and reflect upon one good thing that came from the loss you described previously. How has Jesus been your comforter and healer through this?

CHAPTER 3

Life is an Altar, Not an Idol

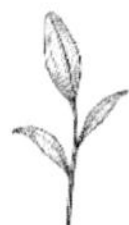

For three years, the depression ebbed and flowed. It came and went as the tides do, pulled by mysterious and invisible forces. When it lapped at the shore of my soul, I became like a hibernating animal, a bear sleeping through winter. The cooling of my emotions and lessening of my willpower brought awareness to this change. All physical processes in me slowed to conserve energy. My cave allowed me to eat little, sleep excessively, and hide from the world. It seemed to turn without me just fine, so it was easy to miss a season or two or three. I woke up, only sporadically and briefly, when the danger of being found out was near.

TIME MACHINE

So that was the goal—to keep this recurring darkness a secret! The pain it caused me encouraged me to prevent it from hurting anyone else. My parents were already overwhelmed with sickness and its effects. How could I add to their stress and trouble? It would also be just as difficult to bear the weight of unwanted scrutiny and attention. Could I really subject myself to more questions and opinions amid all my currently incessant ones? After sifting through the possibilities, I determined the problem was better kept concealed. And perhaps I was better off alone.

Academic, athletic, and social obligations were upheld to very specific standards to maintain the appearance of well-being. Previously, I had been a high achiever with many friends, so I exhausted myself doing whatever it took to discourage suspicion that something might be wrong. Straight A's, starting rosters, and the occasional night out were all strategically earned, attained, or planned. I knew the obvious signs and symptoms of depression and did everything in my power to internalize them. If they showed up in my behavior too much, my determined mission to hide would be sabotaged.

Sometimes, the mask of normalcy would slip after I stretched myself too thin, and certain people noticed. Teachers, coaches, and unrelated parents would ask, "Are you okay? You look a little down."

I always replied, "Yes, I'm good," or "Fine, just tired." These were automatic responses that came out of my mouth without thinking. I truly appreciated their concern, but never saw this question as an opportunity to share honestly. It was simply a cue to shove the pain further down and hide better.

Living that way, surviving in misery, had a way of distorting my perception of time. I was always looking forward and never intentionally present.

- I *mused*, "By the end of this soccer season, I'll be able to relax and recover."
- I *reasoned*, "If I can get through this school year, everything else will be easy."
- I *concluded*, "Once this depressive episode is over, I'll finally have the energy to improve my situation."

Each time I thought this way, it resulted in disappointment. Relaxation, recovery, ease, energy, or improvement never showed up for long before I had to tackle the next obstacle. School years came and went. Birthdays were celebrated. Seasons changed. But I stayed the same.

GOOD CHANGE

Around the age of 15, discussions about moving to a warmer climate intensified. Dad's health was improving, but not enough. He suffered through every Midwestern autumn and winter. The pain worsened, and new symptoms kept coming. It became a matter of life or death again. So, we considered places like Florida, Georgia, and Texas. Must-haves included not only milder weather but also ample job opportunities for Mom. We had a heritage in South Texas, family still living in the area, plenty of economic growth, and it was hot! We took a trip down to visit, and then the final decision was made to leave for good the following summer.

Although stressful, preparing for the move brought me hope. Saying goodbye to everyone and everything I'd ever known was easier than expected. It was decided I could be homeschooled, which was a huge emotional relief. The energy previously spent pretending to be well could now be used more efficiently in actively trying to get well. The time saved by foregoing traditional school would grant me more freedom, which I craved. There would be an entire city with a completely new culture to see and experience. Overall, I was confident that whatever awaited regarding this move had to be better than the last three years of loneliness and monotony.

The new environment was exciting and energizing at first! Exploring the much wider variety of food, shopping, and entertainment was invigorating. The influence of Mexican and cowboy cultures captivated me with their warmth, hospitality, and brightness. I lost myself in new tastes, smells, and sights.

My mind was stimulated, and my interests sparked again. The inspiration that came with encountering such a freshness of life was impossible to ignore. It awakened the creative parts of me I had thought were extinct. However, it quickly sank in that this wasn't a vacation. This was a permanent relocation I was expected to adjust to.

BAD CHANGE

This vibrant but unfamiliar city would have to become more than just a fun place to visit; it would have to become my home. Routines needed to be established, relationships planted, and purposes revealed. I made a sincere effort to discover these things that would bring lasting connection, but I was met with opposition. I joined a soccer club but wasn't accepted as a valuable member of the team. Despite excelling at homeschooling, the lack of supportive friends turned it into a chore. My parents were healthier and happier, but my secret struggle prevented us from rekindling a close relationship.

I still believed that my circumstances must improve subjectively. My thoughts turned to how a place tailored to my sensitivities would alter everything.

- *If my teammates were nicer and more welcoming, then I wouldn't want to quit the team.*
- *If the schools in Texas weren't so enormous, then I might have been brave enough to make some friends.*
- *If my mom and dad hadn't been distracted by health and money, then maybe I could have been more honest.*

But the people, places, and things around me weren't the problem. The problem was my attitude. The book of 1 Thessalonians describes how to hold on to peace and joy no matter what unfolds:

> Rejoice always, pray continually,
> give thanks in all circumstances;
> for this is God's will for you in Christ Jesus.
> 1 THESSALONIANS 5:16–18, NIV

Instead of searching for a silver lining each day and living gratefully in God's grace, I took solace in self-pity and condemned myself to isolation. The cycle of dread and sadness had trapped me once again.

Searching for happiness rather than joy and finding neither, depression and anxiety swelled. In place of the version of myself who once yearned for color and light was a listless stranger. For another two years, my soul blackened and hardened.

My mind proved callous and numb. My will held no power nor discipline. My emotions became violent and unpredictable.

Not only did I have no friendships, but there also seemed to be a long list of people ready and able to injure me. Paranoia of rejection and ridicule prevented me from conversing with others. I rarely spoke to anyone but myself, reverting even further inward, not going out unless forced. Even then, nothing could capture or maintain my interest because it wasn't relatable to the bleakness of my perspective.

FANTASY AND IMAGINATION

Eventually, I turned to idealism and escapism to fill the gaps in my dissatisfaction. Imitations of all the essential human experiences absent in my life could be found in movies, television, and books. My inability to face the fear of rejection and ridicule held me captive, so I ignored and avoided it. There didn't appear to be any point in exploring a dangerous world when a simulation of it could be experienced risk-free. I convinced myself that any real friends or genuine connections were unnecessary—the characters in these fictitious stories would be enough for now.

Whatever conflict was introduced, by the end, it would be settled. Bella Swan received immortality, Rachel Green caught her lobster, and Alice finally found her way back to the riverbank from Wonderland. In the timelines of their stories, it may have taken these protagonists months or years to reach their destinations, but for me, it took mere hours. The faster and more I watched and read, so too did some semblance of order and resolution come to me, even if it was false and temporary.

Unfortunately, this time spent diving into imaginary world after imaginary world was not harmless for me. Indulging in these dramatic narratives offered comfort and safety in fictitious, guaranteed outcomes. These stories had already been curated before they were released. There could be no unexpected change or revision to anything since it had been previously established at some point. The real world—my world—didn't work that way. At any moment, the rug could be pulled out from under my feet, and I would be left reeling for stability again.

I became addicted to chasing what the world of fantasy had to offer: control, perfection, and unlimited potential. Unbeknownst to me, this was a serious problem and prevented me from participating in any present or intentional activity worth doing. It wasn't a question of "What should I do today?" It was a question of, "What should I envision today?" Discomfort and discontent appeared everywhere, triggering my brain to run for its happy place, which was an island of delusion. There was no in-between, no balance, and certainly no moderation, only dwelling in the past or romanticizing the future.

My imagination could have been worth pursuing if it had connected me back to the truth. Like Alice, in my musings, I might have realized there was a home and belonging worth being present for. However, placing my faith in fantasy continued to blur the lines of reality. My unabashedly maximalist ideals and dreams became actual possibilities in my head.

- I *predicted:* One day, I will be a person of real importance.
- I *ascertained:* One day, I will have a partner who worships me.
- I *believed:* One day, my life will be perfect.

This misguided concept of a worldly redemptive "one day" stole any opportunity for spiritual redemption in the present. As beings bound by the constraints of time that God has set, people can only be truly active in the present moment. An individual existed in the past and will exist in the future, but any attempt to direct one's presence apart from the here and now is a form of idolatry. Only God is self-existent and self-sufficient. Engaging in escapism and idealism, I told God whatever He had for me, and whenever it was to be, it wasn't enough.

I would resist and oppose the Lord's plans to correct and restore me at every turn. My opposition to His ultimate purpose for my life, even through this season, simply delayed the inevitable. If He had people lined up to help and encourage me, I never gave them the chance. If He blessed me with favor and hope, I never had the eyes to see it. My self-made altar to revere, honor, and worship imagination drastically inflated my significance and woefully deflated God's. Who was I to tell God He wasn't enough? Merely a liar.

DESPERATE FOR CONTROL

Every social situation, public or private, I visualized beforehand according to my own inclinations and preferences. To anticipate any expectations placed on me, I always asked the *who, what, when* questions. Trips to the mall, meals eaten out, even the shortest of conversations and interactions were rehearsed meticulously. This was not only to maintain a sense of control but also to present an untarnished self-image. I strove to appear as confident and composed as possible.

This thought process was undoubtedly a manifestation of my anxiety. Still, it also became a source of delusional entertainment and fulfillment. It wasn't just about preparing for the worst, but also a confused effort to relate to my surroundings. I simply was not brave enough to be myself, so when disappointment inevitably struck, I created a new version of events in my head.

- There were no awkward silences. I commanded the conversation!
- There were no puzzled looks. Everyone stared at me in awe!
- I wasn't overlooked or forgotten. I belonged somewhere better!

Being able to control others' feelings and perceptions of me, although made-up, meant I could never be misunderstood, disliked, or thought strange. This quickly replaced any wish for a real and meaningful connection. It also gave my heart and mind the freedom to go wild with desire and expectation. When these exaggerated and unrealistic desires and expectations went unmet (which was almost always), I got angry, frustrated, panicked, enraged, and lashed out at anyone around.

It got so bad that chinks in my man-made armor appeared increasingly. I couldn't order a meal at a restaurant or face a cashier. Eye contact with anyone unfamiliar or unknown was out of the question. On multiple occasions, a stranger would speak to me directly, without prior knowledge of my handicap, and receive no answer. All I could do was stare blankly, too frozen to reply or even think of a reply. It was embarrassing and humiliating.

My attempts at controlling the uncontrollable to avoid discord, in fact, led me straight to it. This fated outcome tightened fear's grip around me and introduced agoraphobia. There was no option other than to eliminate the contingencies and liabilities threatening me. It would be infinitely easier and less stressful to stay home and be alone. These practices of idealism and visualization, in which I was the director of events, left no room for anyone else's direction, including God's.

AMBITION AND CONTRIBUTION

Eventually, an opportunity came to join a local teen art class, which helped me regain some normalcy. The art world, which accepted and celebrated free-thinking and rule-breaking, could have led me further astray from God. However, He protected me. In His hands, I could compare different ways of thinking and believing without sacrificing any truly important convictions.

Sharpening my skills and learning techniques held more interest than attempting to establish deeper meaning in my artwork. I had been starved of hands-on experience for quite some time. It was refreshing and revitalizing to again be surrounded by flesh and blood, color and light, and objective cause and effect. Mixing blue and yellow on the palette would always make green. Gradually, I was able to get back to an average level of social skills and even make a few friends.

Throughout those teenage years, I, along with everyone else, was encouraged to select a general professional trajectory. The elementary question, "What do you want to be when you grow up?" evolved into, "Where will you go to university?" and "What will you major in?" I was certainly feeling the increasing pressure to muster up a plan, or at least an answer, for obtaining a useful and productive career. Yet, my underdeveloped brain and my immature heart could decide nothing concrete. The prospect of deciding something so big, so soon, left me unshakably hesitant and cautious.

One day, my father and I discussed the matter and my complete uncertainty about it all, and my resignation to choosing something financially stable. I figured he'd be pleased by my rational side, but he got a far-off look in his eyes.

"Don't ever let things like money or time get in the way of doing what you're called to do," he said. Knowing how he had struggled to find purpose himself, I took his words to heart that day. However pointless it seemed, I muddled through my junior and senior years. Then the time came to make a final decision on further education. The possibilities still appeared endless to me.

- Doctor
- Professor
- Counselor
- Veterinarian
- And so on

I could see myself enjoying and excelling in these professions, but they would also require significant dedication and training. Whatever my choice, there was no guarantee I'd cross the finish line. I certainly hadn't crossed many before.

Thinking ahead (*way* too far ahead), all these unanswerable questions came.

- Could I persevere through all the required schooling?
- If I made it through school, could I then manage the stress of the job?
- If I could manage the stress, for how long would it be sustainable?
- If I found sustainability, would I also find satisfaction?

The idea of again trudging through something that would have permanent effects on my quality of life bred self-doubt. I believed that, somehow, I might find purpose in art, but I couldn't figure out how to turn that into a career. My father's seemingly conflicting advice left me torn. "Sometimes we have to do things we don't want to do," and "Don't let anything get in the way of a calling."

Failing was a great fear that possessed me. Avoiding challenges became a habit to protect against humiliation or disgrace, because I would rather stand quietly than fall loudly. Many family members around me set out on specific paths and accomplished impressive feats. Although I logically understood this required great discipline, it also appeared effortless. They knew what they wanted, determined a way in which to get it, and after some time, it was done.

Between my lack of willpower and inability to see the forest for the trees, neutrality seemed to be the best option. Decisions like these were too important for someone like me, insecure and inflexible, to make. So, either for fear of failure or lack of direction, any aims for college were averted. I decided to play it safe, continue living at home, and find an entry-level job instead.

PROGRESS AND PROFICIENCY

While my job search began, my parents moved away temporarily, and my older sister, Victoria, moved in with me. After weeks of applying anywhere and everywhere, the stakes steadily rising, I finally landed an interview at a craft store. Arriving 30 minutes early, I sat in the car, trembling and buzzing, before mustering up the courage to go in. Submitting myself to this circumstance was nerve-wracking, but my fears were relieved when they offered me a position as a sales associate/cashier.

The tension and stress to impress lifted and were replaced with genuine excitement to get out in the world and leave a mark! I was excited to meet new people and push myself even further. Even though it was a much smaller step than those of my peers, who were heading off to universities, it felt right for me. My efforts to remain neutral and avoid a decision led me to one all the same. This choice would have lasting effects on my life, whether or not I realized it at the time.

There certainly couldn't have been a better way to overcome social anxiety! It was no accident that the only opportunity for work afforded to me was a position in customer service. Every three to five minutes, I was forced to smile and speak cordially to a fresh face. That first day, my heart was pounding! I might have shriveled up and died on the spot if I hadn't known to lean on the Lord for strength. Over and over, my silent plea was, "Help me, God."

How generous and faithful is He who answers every call for help, no matter how small. He shattered my lenses of fear and replaced them with lenses of love. Not only was I finally able to talk to strangers again, but the ability to serve others with kindness and understanding blossomed.

Thanks to Providence, after two weeks, the store manager noticed my remarkable improvements and offered me a new, better position in the art-framing department.

Pushing through social discomfort and inner turmoil meant doing something difficult and inconvenient. Reaping the rewards of perseverance led me one step closer to a potential future in creativity. The two pieces of advice my father gave me no longer clashed. It became clear to me that passion, too, can encounter obstacles. That was not a reason to give in, but a reason to stay determined and remain faithful.

The framing department was always where God intended to put me, but He hadn't handed it to me on a silver platter. He had made me work for it. Not only did it breed resilience within me, but it also protected me from myself. If I had been thrust into this position from the start, I would have failed miserably and been worse off. He gave me time, opportunity, and points of connection to explore and grow into. As a result, my social limits stretched even more, which allowed me to create some lasting friendships.

Things were going really well until the depression returned. By this point, it should have been expected, but it still felt like a major setback. I questioned the worth of my accomplishments before remembering how much progress I'd made recently. That motivated me to keep moving forward. Instead of wallowing, I decided to try out some practical strategies to improve even more!

I figured running, eating, and working would keep the depression away. There would be no more skipping meals or laziness on days off. Although I found some relief, it turned out to be temporary. Soon after implementing these adjustments, my willpower and my commitment to a relationship with God fell through. I didn't even think about asking for His wisdom, direction, or guidance anymore.

I had made an idol of many things, including:

- Time
- Circumstance
- Fantasy
- Control
- Goals
- Progress

Yet, the highest of all these idols was ME.

DESIRES OF THE HEART

As I matured into a woman, incessant loneliness returned to remind me of my deep-set desire for marriage. Friends were great to have, but I certainly couldn't marry them. A profound hunger for emotional intimacy and closeness gripped me. An intense thirst for vulnerability and honesty pursued me. There was one person with whom I could find these experiences in safety and security, and he would be my future husband.

Could these experiences be found, or at least paralleled, in a relationship with Christ?

Yes, but they weren't. Year after year, praying fervently, the Lord sent sign after sign that His promise of marriage was true. Instead of clinging to that promise and waiting patiently for God's timing to be perfect, I clung to my delusions. Picturing a rosy future with Prince Charming took up far too much of my time and energy.

Although there was plenty of internal romantic activity within me at the time, nothing came to fruition. There was no dating. There were no emotionally or physically intimate encounters or relationships. An attraction would reveal itself to be fleeting and superficial at the first exchanged words or shortly after. Every man who could spark any interest at all ended up making me uncomfortable. *It just didn't feel right,* I would think.

This pattern of disappointment should have brought me back to the Lord in humility. It should have led to a conviction from the Holy Spirit, and further, a correction.

- *Stop idealizing men, Elizabeth. How can I prepare you for one husband while you prepare yourself for a hundred husbands?*
- *How can I answer a prayer for a love connection while you ignore opportunities for connection with me, the definition of love?*

Proverbs warns us to keep our hearts in check.

> Above all else, guard your heart,
> for everything you do flows from it.
> PROVERBS 4:23, NIV

I gave my heart too much freedom, and it ran with reckless abandon.

All the stories and scenarios I made up in my head were siphoned from my sometimes deceitful, dangerously powerful heart. If my eyes had been opened to the harm these habits caused, I might also have seen the idolatry, which is replacing God in His rightful position with something else. Guessing, estimating, overthinking, and fabricating placed *me* where *God* should be.

The only altars in existence should be to our God, who is the self-existent origin of everything, throughout and outside of time. I was building altars for everyone and everything but Him. Instead of turning to God as father, friend, and partner, I turned further into myself, even going so far as seeking a position above Him.

Certainly, these unsavory and unwise mental practices caused my depression and anxiety to worsen even further.

REFLECTION AND CORRECTION

Life is an Altar, Not an Idol

Although most idols in the Bible were statues, totems, and talismans made of metal, stone, and wood, anything worshiped in place of God can be an idol.

> But their idols are silver and gold, made by human hands.
> They have mouths, but cannot speak, eyes but cannot see.
> They have ears, but cannot hear, noses, but cannot smell.
> They have hands, but cannot feel, feet, but cannot walk,
> Nor can they utter a sound with their throats.
> Those who make them will be like them,
> And so will all who trust in them.
>
> PSALM 115:4–8, NIV

Common forms of idolatry today (aside from statues, totems, and talismans, which still exist) include physical satisfaction (food and sex), materialism (money and possessions), and vanity (image and status).

I myself have idolized time, circumstance, fantasy, control, ambition, progress, and desire.

Fill out the following chart to reveal: What have you idolized, previously or currently? What did/does your worship of these idols look like? How would your worship change if these idols were replaced with an intentional and wholehearted relationship with God?

IDOL	IDOLIC WORSHIP	GODLY WORSHIP
E.g., Money	Working 7 days per week	Sabbath rest 1 day per week

Life is not meant to be the object of your worship, an idol. Life is a means for you to worship God, an altar.

Whatever pleasure, provision, or prosperity we receive from the idols we make will never be enough in their temporary forms. Everlasting pleasure, provision, and prosperity can only be received in eternal life through Jesus Christ.

Set your minds on things above, not on earthly things.
For you died and your life is now hidden with Christ in God.
When Christ, who is your life, appears,
then you will also appear with him in glory.
COLOSSIANS 3:2–4, NIV

PART TWO:

THE BATTLE

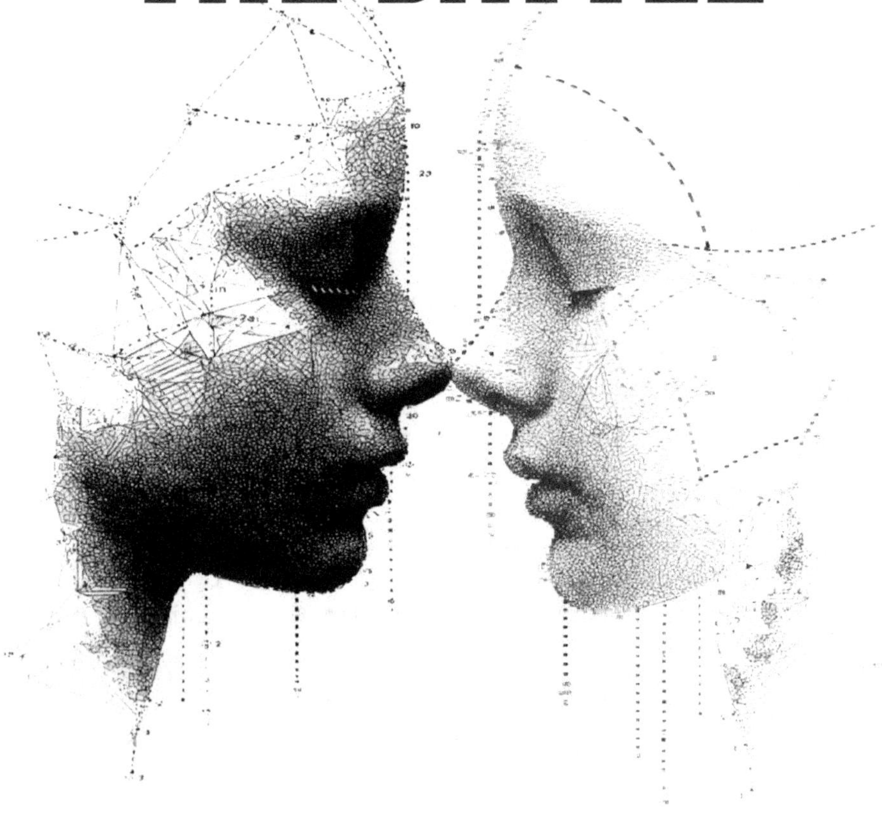

CHAPTER 4

Jesus Paid it All

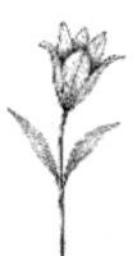

By now, I had endured six cycles of depression, ranging from a few months to over a year, and each episode was worse than the last. Familiarity can provide a sense of comfort, even in misery. Depression over the years had become all too familiar and oh-so comfortable, which made it that much easier to welcome the gloom whenever it returned.

ANOTHER MOUNTAIN CLIMBED

It wasn't a slow, gentle slope anymore but a fast, jarring drop-off. Without understanding what had occurred or why, I looked up from a new rock bottom, no closer to finding answers than before. Detached indifference ground away at my psyche like sandpaper. It dulled my personality to bluntness and propelled me further into darkness.

Repeated trials, endless toil, and countless climbs led only to failure after failure, leaving me exhausted and desperate. Any effort to find relief from the vicious cycles of depression and the unpredictable challenges of mental instability seemed in vain. Even though I achieved some success in easing my anxiety through practical methods, sadness and unfulfillment persisted. Any progress proved pointless without:

- The capacity to continue improving,
- Enough endurance and willpower to implement said improvements, and
- The motivation and desire to choose progress in the first place.

How many more attacks of hopelessness could I endure before I lost my mind entirely?

ANOTHER PLATEAU HIT

My nineteenth birthday brought me to a point of reflection. I mused over the years leading up to that day and realized something had to give. A mysterious inner struggle had consumed my relatively short life. I thought, "How long should I go on dreaming and waiting for nothing? What if there's more? There *has* to be more." A rare flash of optimism encouraged me to believe that happiness surely couldn't evade me forever.

I decided—then and there—that depression wouldn't ruin my future. A sudden determination came upon me. "Enough is enough!" Despite my past failures, I could not be convinced to give up hope yet. But, no matter what I tried or for how long, it seemed this evil could not be banished by my efforts alone. The depression would not budge long-term, a problem requiring help beyond myself. What else was there to try but medical intervention?

It seemed clear that seeking professional assistance might be the one thing I was missing all along. Although my previously practical methods for achieving balance were valuable and constructive, I lacked the motivation to maintain them consistently. These efforts were sporadic and, many times, half-hearted. I lacked the self-discipline and self-control to finish what was started and remain consistent in any endeavors to improve. Despite deliberately avoiding the world of modern medicine for so long, I was tired of feeling trapped.

It's possible my judgment was clouded by the intense longing to win this mental war. Maybe I gave in too soon and didn't exhaust all the other options. Regardless of my failure to understand, God would certainly be with me. The Holy Spirit was working within to make a move that would bring me back into alignment with Him. The winds of change were palpable, an eerie premonition of the subtle yet significant shifts that would soon reveal themselves.

IN THE PALM OF GOD'S HANDS

My choice to ask for help that day would forever alter my life. I started on the middle ground with every intention of rising higher. But I would first be taken so low, lower than I ever thought possible. What was to come or how God planned to use it was unclear, but a message from the book of Isaiah added a piece to that puzzle.

"For my thoughts are not your thoughts,
neither are your ways my ways," declares the LORD.
"As the heavens are higher than the earth,
so are my ways higher than your ways
and my thoughts than your thoughts."

ISAIAH 55:8–9, NIV

I would encounter powerful evil and terrible lies, but God would carry me through. There could be no valley beyond His reach. He masterfully and mysteriously guided me exactly to where I needed to be. Not only was this for my benefit, but also for the benefit of others. My loving creator effortlessly orchestrated every person, place, and event to guide me back to His truth and love. Who else but someone all-knowing and all-present could paint a masterpiece such as this?

TAKING THE FIRST STEP

The process was initially straightforward. My mother, now a nurse practitioner, offered a personal referral to a doctor she knew. Some might assume the referral would have been to a psychiatrist or mental health specialist. However, it was decided that primary care would suffice, because we believed all I needed was an antidepressant. Medicine alone should be enough to get me back on track.

Even though the clinic was an hour away, I scheduled the appointment and made the commute because my family trusted this doctor. It was a big step to take and a huge commitment to make for someone who still struggled with anxiety. Being alone in the car allowed me to prepare and gather my thoughts before the social interaction (Perhaps some introverts would appreciate that sentiment!).

It went just as expected. The office atmosphere was as warm and welcoming as a sterile healthcare facility could be. The nurse asked me basic health questions and took my vital signs, while the doctor gained my trust.

Dr. Kelly was a colleague of my mother's and my father's provider amid his many health problems. So, it made sense that he would be friendly, personable, and genuinely concerned for me.

It was reassuring to know he had a deeper understanding of my struggle because of his prior knowledge of my circumstances. His promise—even if it was through legal obligation—to not share any information with my parents without my consent sealed my trust in him. My parents knew that I had been fighting mentally and mostly losing. The struggles were hard to miss, but they did not know specific details.

Every effort to shield them was rooted in fearing an exacerbation of their pain and distress and their potential interference. Their intervention wouldn't be the end of the world, but I'd lose the little control I possessed. Dr. Kelly seemed impartial and discreet. God knew these characteristics would be valuable, not only for this visit but also for more challenging future ones.

The same standard protocols and policies applied to patients seeking care for depression also applied to me. Soon enough, the question was asked, "Over the last two weeks, how often have you been bothered by any of the following problems:

- Finding little interest or pleasure in doing things?
- Feeling down or hopeless?
- Having trouble staying asleep or sleeping too much?
- Having little energy, poor appetite, or overeating?
- Feeling bad about yourself?
- Experiencing trouble concentrating or completing tasks?
- Considering thoughts that you would be better off dead or hurting yourself?"

Most of my answers to these questions were "more than half the days per week" and "nearly every day". Obviously, this was not news to me. I had completed twenty or more of these questionnaires online for the past six years, with very similar results. While I was already aware of my current depression, establishing a baseline was crucial for Dr. Kelly to track my progress. Ideally, the frequency and severity of these problems would decrease as the medicine did its job.

Seeing these signs and symptoms listed so plainly on a piece of paper felt surreal. The painful presence of how much joy and experience had been robbed from me was stark. There could not have been a more irrelevant and impersonal phrase than "over the last two weeks" throughout the questionnaire. Sure, it was just a general term to represent continuity over time, but for me, two weeks passed in the blink of an eye. Two weeks had passed before they began. Two weeks felt as empty as the same old mistakes and the same old promises I'd made to myself over the last seven years!

Seven years going through cycle after cycle of depression with very little normalcy in between. I envied those who could find themselves in the phrase "over the last two weeks" and wondered how many people found themselves better suited to "over the past few decades." Like many people, I had wasted an exponential amount of time on the enemy's schemes of confusion, sorrow, and bitterness. Illustrated with ink, it would blot out most of my existence. When seasons change, there's a tendency to mourn what's left behind; in my case, I mourned what never was.

CONTINUING IN UNCERTAINTY

With the support of my parents and Dr. Kelly, I accepted this new path. His first suggestion was to try Prozac or generic fluoxetine. However, following a previous conversation with my mother, we chose Zoloft, or sertraline. Both drugs were selective serotonin reuptake inhibitors, or SSRIs. SSRIs treat depression by increasing levels of serotonin in the brain and blocking its reabsorption, thus improving the brain's ability to send messages. I had minimal knowledge about the medication, except for a preconceived notion that it was generally safe because of its widespread use.

Dr. Kelly reiterated that the medicine would need time to take effect and advised me to practice patience. I resigned myself to a few more weeks of melancholy to ultimately find a remedy. Throughout the appointment, he offered comfort and expressed relief at my search for aid, reassuring me of his confidence in my ability to receive it.

Making strong eye contact, he said, "We're going to get you the help that you need."

Although emotionally and mentally drained after the appointment, I believed the worst was over. The medication was collected a few days later. Yet, I was oblivious to the immeasurable darkness that would arise from such a small bottle of pills.

FALLING FAST

Despite the possibility that positive results would be slow to arrive, Dr. Kelly reassured me that improvement would come. But it never did. Days went by, but I did not feel better. Weeks went by, but I did not feel better. One month passed—still no advance in recovery.

In fact, due to a sharp mental decline, Dr. Kelly discontinued my use of Zoloft and prescribed Prozac instead. Unfortunately, the switch in medication did nothing to reverse my negative trajectory.

Quietly and quickly, "no better" transitioned into "*much, much* worse." I was unaware of the medicine's injury, being blinded by its guises and numb to its severity. It all happened so fast, there was no time to process the darkness that had come to ravage me again. Only after my actions proved the buried intuition inside did I wake from the chemical stupor. Then a great season of sin and shame began, which some readers may relate to.

BLOOD

I started cutting myself. The specifics of my first self-inflicted wound or its location are unclear. What sticks is the cool steel of the razor blade between my thumb and pointer finger. The line turned from translucent to red, accompanied by a sting and then burning. Initially, the habit was adopted with caution, but its intensity and recklessness escalated daily.

Like many others, the primary goal of this self-harm was not to injure myself seriously, but to defy the apathy forced upon me by depression. Regardless of my misguided intentions, this was a level of evil I'd never known, and it took me to impossible depths of despair and depravity. With no feelings besides torment and anguish to tether me to the life I once lived, I was barely existing.

Continuing to feed this hunger for blood gave me hope it would soon be satiated. However, the addiction to the pain grew. Through consistent practice, a balance was struck between gratification and maintaining made-up boundaries of comfort and safety. I would test how much pressure was too much pressure and experiment with slow incisions versus fast incisions. If the skin was pulled taut, my blows were swift and concise enough to pacify the urge. This was how far I had fallen: contemplating all the gory details of which strategy reigned supreme in marking my flesh and finding fulfillment in performing it well.

Of course, my audience remained unseen. Ironically, even though this was the darkest time in my life, I remained oblivious to the spiritual presence of evil. You'd think I'd have known my demons by name because they never left my side. Surely, the seriousness of my actions in shedding the blood and mutilating the flesh of a body bought and paid for would've hit me.

Those demons were saying, "We may not have her eternity, but look how she forsakes you now." They reveled in the perversion. They delighted in my actions, which mocked the perfect and pure sacrifice of Jesus Christ.

It is a tool of the enemy to reveal themselves only when it's convenient and helpful to them. Demons had no problem making scary faces in my nightmares as a child. But when it came time for blood rituals, their likeness stayed hidden in the shadows.

Now, I realize the cowardice and selfishness of their nature. A smug voice comes to me amid this reflection, saying, "Remember when you mutilated your flesh for me?" It's quite a revelation that the enemy confessed to being complicit in crimes like mine.

TRUTH AND GRACE

If I'd been more conscious of the spiritual conflict, I might have embraced good, light, and love rather than evil, darkness, and hate. A passage in Romans declares the undying and unfailing love of Christ that I could have held onto.

> But God demonstrates his own love for us in this:
> while we were still sinners, Christ died for us.
> ROMANS 5:8, NIV

If His love for me did not falter on the cross, how could it ever falter?

When His head was crowned with thorns, His love never failed.

When His hands and feet were pierced with nails, His love never failed.

When He cried out through His last breath, His love never failed.

Another presence also comes to me—a silent presence, not from lack of feeling or words, but from a surplus of unspeakable sorrow. Oh, how my actions saddened the Lord. Oh, how it pained Him to watch me partake in such evil. While the enemy revealed his presence, the Lord's presence revealed the truth. God wasn't watching me with a scornful and judgmental eye. He was watching me through the lens of His love, which defeats sin and transcends understanding. He didn't shake His head and turn away. He stayed and felt my own physical and emotional pain alongside me. For every tear I shed, He shed ten thousand more.

God knows exactly how many cuts I made, how many faded, and how many scarred. Still, that number is zero compared to the power of His redemption. His love for me remained the same, despite my deep offenses against Him. I purposely and perversely shed the blood He placed in my veins for His glory, yet when I asked for forgiveness, it was already there, whole and free.

God shows the depth and magnitude of sin not to condemn, but to align our hearts with His heart, which is pure and holy. Correction of the heart leads to correction of action, which is true repentance. Only the love of Jesus Christ could overcome my guilt and shame.

Of course, there is no sin that does not warrant death. If I had gossiped, murdered, stolen, or lied, I would deserve nothing less than death. While externally harming myself with a blade was especially heinous, my daily sins caused internal harm all the same. Evil is evil, no matter what form it takes. Consequences and punishments may vary in degree, but sin is sin, and its final wage is death. The point of this is not condemnation, but glorification of the God who forgives all. Romans further explains that even though humans deserve Hell, God wants to give us Heaven.

For the wages of sin is death,
but the gift of God is eternal life in Christ Jesus our Lord.

ROMANS 6:23, NIV

Through holy justification, no one is defined by their past, present, or future sins. One who is saved by grace, through faith, is declared righteous even in the midst of unrighteousness. I deserved death, and still deserve death, yet He gave me life. God saw past my sin and straight into me, someone worth saving. This gift alone should have been enough of an invitation to return to Him, no matter how hard it was.

Sadly, I did not have the enlightened perspective back then that I cling to now. While grasping the seriousness of my deteriorating mental state, this practice of shedding blood continued. Before long, I ran out of room. My arms, legs, sides, hips, and chest were all occupied with notches. It became uncomfortable to sleep because of the painful pressure on my wounds while lying down. However, even pain was a sort of comfort. These stinging sensations kept me from losing my grip on reality. It truly was a season of shame—the greatest season of shame in my life—yet God was with me.

THE ENEMY'S MISSION

Shame is another tool the enemy uses. Despite knowing it was wrong, the shame of the sins I'd fallen into kept me from stopping. How could I return to a perfect and holy Father as an imperfect and unholy daughter? I couldn't shake off the disgrace of my actions despite my faith and encounters with God's forgiveness. The knowledge was buried and hidden.

The enemy reminded me of my sin daily, and I believed the lie that I was unredeemable. Evil spirits shoved their way into my heart and mind with their intrusive and violent accusations. These were the thoughts assigned to me:

- *I am too broken.*
- *I am not good enough.*
- *I am unworthy.*

Believing their lies trapped me in a prison of guilt and unworthiness. If the enemy's mission was destruction, then his greatest success would be found in death, the ultimate form of destruction. Many times, I wished for my life to be taken, even ludicrously praying God Himself would take me. The medication had built up in my system. It altered my brain chemistry and dissolved my discernment.

Cutting my way through so many standards of righteousness made righteousness itself seem to be a made-up construct. If I wanted to die, then why couldn't I? Surely my suffering deserved mercy. God hadn't appeared merciful to me lately, anyway. It took incredible courage to reach out for help, yet I'd been dropped into a pit of snakes, each fighting for a bite of my soul. How could I continue in such misery?

For the first time, instead of just wondering and wishing, I started planning. The boundary was broken. Life held no meaning. What would be the easiest and most efficient way to die? I could not subject my family to any extremely violent method nor risk poison failing. I had no idea how difficult it was to decide matters of death until attempting to plan my own.

Finally ready to give up after what felt like a lifetime of struggle, and even that seemed impossible! With no solid options, I hoped my newly developed and shockingly violent impulses would eventually decide for me. Regardless of how it happened, the day would come soon, and it would be over. There was no visible light; only darkness, with no hope for a life worth living.

One evening, in the confines of my black hole of a bedroom, I succumbed to the voices pushing me to seize control of my destiny. My sole personal space was in a disastrous state, mirroring my mind and goading me even further in my impulses. The last straw was my continual failure to keep my room tidy. Something so simple convinced me I was a complete and utter failure.

Slumped on the floor, surrounded by piles of clothing and trash, I spotted a scarf within arm's reach. It was in a gray animal print, probably a hand-me-down, and it was soft in my hands. Staring at it for so long, time seemed to stand still. Wondering if it would feel just as soft wrapped around my neck, I put it on just like the last twenty times, with a double loop, but with different intentions.

Just try it.

The tighter I pulled, the further the pressure spread, warm and welcoming.

Just see how far you can go.

Pulling it even tighter stole my ability to breathe. I kept pulling. Blood was not enough; they were greedy for my breath, too, and I was ready to relinquish it.

It is a myth that one cannot commit self-strangulation. Maybe that's why there was no sense of urgency to stop. Despite my lungs burning dry and my vision turning black, I pulled tighter. The pulling stopped at some point, but I don't have a clear memory of when. Either I passed out, or my arms failed me.

Regardless of the details, it was at that moment that my brokenness hit me. My will, mind, and emotions were shattered and scattered across desolate physical and spiritual landscapes. Nothing was left of my former self except a tiny seed of hope. Remembering the God of my childhood and recalling His love for me, I wept on the floor with a scarf around my neck.

PEACE

The morning light felt like a comforting breath of fresh air. The demons had been held at bay once again, allowing me to make it through another night, barely. My actions the previous evening were unlike anything I had ever experienced. It was frightening. It felt as if someone else had done it, not me. A new sense of urgency to take the situation seriously came over me. I could not continue on this dark path. Another encounter in the night might prove fatal.

Stepping outside onto the warm concrete, I took a deep breath. My lungs filled deeply and slowly while the birds sang. The warmth of the rising sun's rays bathed my arms and face. Lying back and watching the clouds float lazily in the sky reminded me of how God's creation always calmed me.

That beautiful early morning light, after the blackest of nights, grounded me. God had afforded a pocket of peace for me to find rest. The voice of reason had returned. If God's creation of nature, secondary to man, could incite such positivity, then surely, as a primary creation, I could not be as powerless as I believed.

TAKING ANOTHER STEP

The comfort of the natural world and warm sun bolstered my courage to call Dr. Kelly. I was nervous and anxious to speak to him. Although he had already expressed increasing concern, being aware of my tendency to self-harm, revealing even more of what had unraveled behind closed doors, was daunting. It was hard to accept that I'd fallen so far.

Saying it out loud, especially in the presence of another, would make it real. I would no longer be able to pretend I could handle it alone, and everything would be fine. Acknowledging it would force me to face the challenge of bringing this all-too-familiar evil to light. It was another prominent moment in my journey that would stay with me for years. I had already faced many decisions, and this one would not be allowed to haunt me with regret. Taking the next step required me to swallow my pride and fight my fear.

Despite the early hour, he answered, and I communicated my state of crisis in a few words. "Crisis" is more or less a term used to describe when someone's life is at stake—a life-or-death situation. I did not use the words "attempted suicide" because I wasn't sure that truly happened. But I tried my best to express how each day was worse than the last and that I now teetered on the edge of disaster.

Dr. Kelly needed little convincing when I described the events of the previous evening vaguely with phrases like "I crossed a line" and "I'm scared of myself." In fact, he became the convincer. At our previous appointment, he had already suggested that I check myself into the hospital for a higher-level opinion. He repeated this suggestion to me multiple times throughout the phone call, and his tone was concerned and urgent. He was more afraid for me than I was for myself.

While knowing this would likely be his advice, I still hesitated. The possibility of finally getting answers to all my "whys" appealed to me, but fear and cowardice never strayed far. Eventually, he said there wasn't much else he could do. The medication wasn't working as it should, and the situation had grown beyond his depth. I ultimately relented, not only because it was the right choice, but also to appease the man who had tried his very best to help me, with no success.

Agreeing to his proposal required my promise to handle all the preparations for hospital admission. My sister, Victoria, agreed to drive me there. My boss honored my request for a few days off for medical reasons and told me he would pray for me.

Thanks to God, it all went smoothly, without hindrance or hiccup. This was the correct path, even if the reasons were unclear. Soon, everything would make sense.

Over the following days, there was cautious optimism. Working diligently, I prepared myself. Assuredly, the worst had already come to pass, and I'd officially hit rock bottom. But my story didn't end at rock bottom, and to get back on top, I'd have to climb again! There was the casual concern that this next climb would all be for naught, like those of the past. I contemplated what I would have to fix in myself for things to be different. I considered whether whatever God had in store would be worth it. Change is possible, but rarely is it easy or instant.

After the night of the incident, sleeping in my bedroom no longer felt comfortable or safe. I feared and distrusted myself and the dark forces I had encountered. Alone and isolated in my personal space, their influence was strongest. I was sure they couldn't manipulate me further, but their presence was a dangerous temptation, nonetheless. Revisiting the place where they spurred me to attack myself again and again required bravery beyond me. I was not yet strong enough to fight them head-on. Sleeping on the couch warded off their pursuit.

REFLECTION AND CORRECTION

Jesus Paid it All

The topic of sin can be uncomfortable and difficult to face. When we reflect honestly on our thoughts and actions, which we are always accountable for, we are confronted with the magnitude of our fallen nature.

Try to recall the most harmful action you have ever committed.

How did this action negatively affect you and those around you? Do you still harbor any guilt or shame?

____

____

____

____

____

____

When God the Father allowed Jesus Christ to be crucified 2,000 years ago, He knew you would need His grace today! Through repentance, God shows us the cost of our sin. Through forgiveness, God shows us His grace is enough to cover that cost.

Chart 1 below provides examples of sins or debts that come against us. Take notice of the payment status: PAID IN FULL. On Chart 2, write some of your debts and mark them as PAID IN FULL.

DEBT	**STATUS**
Self-Harm	**PAID IN FULL**
Lust	**PAID IN FULL**
Suicidal Ideation	**PAID IN FULL**

CHART 1

DEBT	STATUS

CHART 2

Jesus paid for abortion, homosexuality, abuse, murder, prostitution, addiction, divorce, adultery, and a multitude of other sins. 1 John says this about Jesus:

> He is the atoning sacrifice for our sins,
> and not only for ours but also for the sins
> of the whole world.
>
> 1 JOHN 2:2, NIV

Jesus paid it all. Your sin doesn't make you untouchable. In fact, God sees every single sin inside and out, past, present, and future, and still He offers His spotless hand for you to hold. He sent His Son, Jesus, to pay your debt, already knowing the cost.

No one is so dirty that His mercy cannot cleanse. No one is so broken that His love cannot mend. No one is so lost that His presence cannot find them. **Accept His payment and be free**.

CHAPTER 5

Surrender is Victory

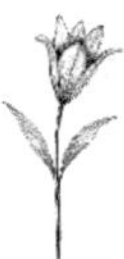

The day finally came to check myself into the hospital. Knowing it must be done didn't change the anxious energy and dread I woke up with. Despite the July heat in Texas, my long sleeves and pants covered my wounds and scars. Each mark was at various stages of healing, some fresh and tender, others dry and itchy.

My clothes painfully rubbed against them, but the idea of bearing my sin on display for the world to see was unthinkable. The shame and guilt made me want to dig myself a hole to hide in, but some people prevented me from grabbing a shovel.

A LEAP OF FAITH

My sister, Victoria, accompanied me to Dr. Kelly's office for one more visit. Once we arrived, no time was wasted. Questionnaires and formalities were forgotten by this point. Dr. Kelly simply wanted to ensure we were all on the same page. He recommended a specific hospital and instructed us to go there immediately. He explained that as soon as I was admitted, an inpatient appointment would be made with a psychiatrist who should have answers. Victoria was solemnly on board, but even after everything, I was still hesitant.

Dr. Kelly must have sensed my trepidation and asked, "How are you feeling about all of this?" It was my last chance to jump ship, and I couldn't stop myself from trying. Tears welling, I told him, "I really don't want to go." He firmly yet delicately expressed that this was absolutely necessary. There was nothing further he could do within his scope of practice, and he couldn't allow me, in good conscience, to continue unsafely. I had a fleeting thought, by the look in his eye, that without my compliance, he might somehow force me to go, anyway.

I was a danger to myself and had all but admitted that to him on multiple occasions in multiple ways. There were rules, policies, and safeguards in place. Reasonable cause for concern that life—either my own or others'—might be taken, qualified for the forfeit of certain rights. Of course, I didn't want to give up my rights or my dignity. But something inside me had already snapped, which caused me to relinquish plenty. Despite wishing it wasn't so, I knew the time for hiding was over.

ASSISTANCE AND ASSURANCE

Victoria and I drove back into the city, stopping for lunch before continuing to the emergency room. She most likely knew from her experience as a nurse that there wouldn't be another opportunity to eat for a while. Perhaps she was also looking for some common ground. We were not terribly close as sisters, but the current situation forced us to face each other without pretense. Sitting across the table from her, eating a tasteless sandwich, heaviness filled the air.

Throughout the meal, I repeatedly expressed my reluctance to go. I longed to run far away where nobody could reach me, as I had for the last seven years. Then Victoria spoke.

"You know that most people never get help? You're doing something that most people in your position never do."

She said this seriously, without blinking. Coming from her, who took after our no-nonsense father, this was a big compliment. I understood that she meant that while this was a hard thing to do, it was also a good thing, and it shut me up.

My sister reminded me of the truth I learned as a little girl: Fear is a liar. My fear might have morphed into a full-blown panic attack had it not been stopped in its tracks. Victoria knew better and would not justify my acting on fear. The time for chasing feelings was over because God was calling me to be brave. Bravery is not the absence of fear, but perseverance through it. No matter what I felt, it must be done. Praise God for orchestrating it just so!

It was not a surprise to God that I would want to back out at the last second. He placed Dr. Kelly and Victoria, two people with vast knowledge and discernment, to prevent me from running away again. He softened and opened their hearts so that I might find help and hope in them. I could not bring myself to say another word about not going to the hospital. The fear and dread in my heart were replaced with peace and submission. We finished eating our food and left for the emergency room.

A COG IN THE MACHINE

When we arrived, it was busy and loud, as emergency rooms in the city usually are. We checked in with a receptionist and found seats between someone coughing behind a mask and another talking loudly on their cellphone. I was grateful for the distractions but anxious to get away from these strangers who created an atmosphere of anonymity. I had come to be seen, but felt lost in that waiting room.

To combat my rising anxiety, I replayed my sister's words and reminded myself that this was a good thing. It was only a matter of time until I felt that goodness, and I needed only to be patient. After over two hours, my name was called, and we headed to a triage area. Scribes and physicians alike, even one on a computer screen, asked the same basic question. "What brought you to the emergency room today?"

Once it was well established that I had come because of suicidal ideation, the questions became more intense, and honesty grew more difficult. I had never met these people and would surely never meet them again. What right did they have to know such deeply personal things about me? Obviously, the cuts, scabs, and scars could not be hidden forever. But I was not about to abandon all sense of self-preservation. I decided to tell them only what they needed to hear to admit me, and not a word more. The conversation went something like this:

"Are you receiving treatment for depression? Is the medication helping?"

"Yes, and no."

"Do you have a plan to end your life?"

A half-truth. "No."

"Have you ever attempted suicide before?"

Another half-truth. "No."

"Are you self-harming?"

"Yes."

"When was the last time you self-harmed?"

"Yesterday."

"Where are the wounds located on your body?"

"Everywhere."

The questioning continued as we were moved from one area of the hospital to the next. Every medical professional had the same questions and came to the same conclusion: I should be admitted for my own safety, but also for further analysis. Psychiatrists were not present in the emergency room, so it became a matter of waiting for a bed on the psych floor to become available. It was currently full. I had to wait for my turn.

In the meantime, they made me change into disposable scrubs, as was policy for all psych patients, because I posed a safety risk to myself and others. All my original clothing and belongings were secured in a plastic drawstring bag. They led me to where my sister already waited, in a room with three other non-psych patients. Our small personal spaces were separated by pleated paper curtains.

My area did not have a bed, only two chairs opposite each other—one for my sister and one for me. There was a large window spanning the entire rectangular room where we could see all the doctors and nurses working. They sat at their computers, inputting information, answering calls, and researching treatments for various conditions. By this time, it was evening. Victoria and I were rightfully exhausted.

WHAT A MESS

I didn't want to think anymore, but being so close to the finish line, the thoughts wouldn't quiet. They fixated on all it took to get to this moment. Choosing to bear depression on my own so many years ago would unknowingly lead me to this place of extreme sickness and desperation. Confessing my shame to so many foreign and detached faces was mortifying. They either stared for too long or barely glanced my way.

Heavy shame, sorrow, and guilt bore down on me for allowing this type of darkness to cultivate in my soul and life.

I'd been wearing black that day, like most days lately, and it was an accurate illustration of my innermost parts. The darkness had almost consumed me, and this day proved that. Now I was curled up in an uncomfortable chair, dressed in polypropylene garments that itched everywhere they touched. I had become so lost, so ugly, and so dead.

After stowing away the pain in a hidden place for almost a decade, something gave way and broke through. It was like the floodgates opened. My body racked itself with sobs, the tears flowed like a river, and the room became silent apart from my cries. For the first time in seven years, I allowed someone to see me cry. Victoria seemed shocked at first, but quickly recovered and moved to cradle me on her lap.

She asked urgently, "What's wrong? What is it? What happened?"

I replied through howls of agony, "I don't know. I don't know. I don't know."

Words of explanation wouldn't form. The room spun, and my heart clenched. My head ached from all the jumbled-up thoughts. Victoria held me like a baby in her arms. She hushed and soothed me while I wailed. It was some time before I could calm down.

Hours later, Victoria expressed that she could no longer stay. We'd been gone all day, and she had to go home to take care of some things, but promised to return. Before leaving, she wrote her and our father's phone numbers on a slip of paper. She instructed me to hold on to it in case I was admitted without her. There were no incoming calls to the psych ward, so it would be up to me to contact them. I placed the scrap in the front pocket of my paper scrubs for safekeeping.

ADMIT ONE 637–2

After even more waiting, finally a nurse came to inform me that a bed on the psychiatric floor had become available. He explained that I would be transported to the appropriate department in a separate building via ambulance. Shortly, two paramedics arrived outside the room with a gurney. I was required to lie down and be strapped in.

They informed me it was standard procedure for all psych patients and not to worry.

We traveled through a few fluorescent-lit hallways and down an elevator before reaching an entrance where the ambulance was parked. They loaded me up, and we drove a very short distance before stopping. After unloading me, we continued down a couple more white hallways leading to another elevator. Finally, they removed my restraints and allowed me to get off the gurney.

One paramedic left the way we came while another escorted me onto the elevator. She also held my bag of belongings. The doors opened to a small, secured area flanked by a set of locked doors. The paramedic buzzed in, and a nurse opened those doors. All the lights were dimmed apart from a central nurse's station. No one was around but me and two nurses. It was silent and still. Then and there, I became a ward of the psychiatric unit.

One nurse took my belongings and transferred them to a paper bag, while the other took my vitals and gave me a wristband. I had a slight fever, which they supposed was from dehydration after we'd been sitting and waiting for over eight hours. One nurse got me a small electrolyte drink, and we continued with the admission process.

I was taken to a small exam room and answered the same questions as before. Only this time, when it came up that I'd been self-harming, they needed to see the wounds. I protested at first, explaining there were too many; I would have to take everything off. The nurse was firm in her request, explaining that lifting each section of clothing one at a time would suffice.

So, I lifted my shirt to show her the marks on my abdomen and chest, then folded down the waist of my pants on each side to reveal the fresh wounds on my hips. Rolling up my sleeves displayed more angry red lines. Lastly, I lifted each pant leg to show her the scabs on my shins and thighs. She glanced at each section briefly, marked the location down on her paper, and that was that.

Then she led me back to the main area and into a room filled with tables and chairs. I sat down with another new face—some sort of admissions worker—to go over my rights, responsibilities, and hospital rules. She also informed me of the daily schedule, including group activities and meals. They needed me to fill out an order for each meal every time I ate.

"You'll probably just get a general breakfast tomorrow until the paperwork goes through," she explained.

Apparently, all of this was of the utmost importance because it couldn't wait until morning. The hospital rules included:

- My right to considerate and respectful care
- My right to request or refuse treatment
- My right to refuse or accept visitors
- No sharp objects of any kind
- No belts, shoelaces, or strings of any kind
- All personal items must be inspected and approved by hospital staff
- Participation in group therapy and activities is highly encouraged
- A psychiatric assessment is required during admission
- Patient must agree to receive continuing healthcare prior to discharge
- Outgoing phone calls are permitted during specific hours
- Visitation is only permitted during specific hours

Next, I was shown to my shared room. There was a tiny, brown-tiled bathroom complete with a shower, sink, and toilet. The rest of it was compact and square, with a large window at the back wall. Two beds and two desks arranged parallel to each other on each side wall were the only furniture. I noticed someone sleeping in the first bed as I was led to my own. The nurse said my roommate's name was Lucy, so I deduced that the heavily breathing form must be her. They gave me a dosage of the sleeping pill trazodone, then I curled up in my hospital bed and fell asleep to the sound of Lucy's breathing.

DAY ONE

In the morning, the sound of footsteps and squeaky metal woke me up. I squinted and peeked above my covers to see a tall man wearing white scrubs stooping beside Lucy's bed. She sighed and extended her wrist-banded arm to him from beneath her blankets. He inserted a needle and extracted some of her blood. I closed my eyes and wondered if this was another standard procedure or something special for Lucy.

I got my answer when the man thanked "Miss Lucy" and rolled his cart over to me. He assumed I was sleeping and whispered, "Miss Elizabeth? I need to see your wristband and take some blood." I complied by sticking out my arm like Lucy. He compared my wristband with his own labels, pierced my skin, and took three vials of blood. Then he said, "Thank you, I'll see you tomorrow. We do this every morning."

Returning to sleep failed as the whirlwind that was yesterday swept through my mind. I hoped that all of this would be worth receiving the answer I'd been looking for. A vision of myself reached for something, stretching out as far as possible, but I managed to fall back asleep before grasping whatever mysterious thing I'd been missing.

More noise woke me up for the second time that day, but it was louder and further away. Nurses spoke to one another, and several people walked up and down the hallway. Metal chair legs scraped across the floor somewhere, and doors opened and closed. Rolling over revealed Lucy's empty bed, neatly made. I was glad she was not there to see me take everything in through the light of day.

It was a relief to be in a place where I could no longer hurt myself or be alone with my demons, but I was also extremely uncomfortable. The hospital was cold and arid; the furnishings and finishes were old and dingy. My only clothes were paper scrubs and grippy socks. I felt groggy and loopy from the sleeping pill the night before as I walked from my room back to the nurse's station.

Looking around, I spotted a familiar space, the room filled with tables and chairs. It turned out to be a dining hall for all the patients on the floor. There were probably 8 to 10 other people eating. Lucy was clearing her tray and leaving, so I took an empty seat and waited for my cafeteria-style breakfast tray. It was not what I ordered, but the lady had told me to expect that. There was also a card to fill out detailing my requests for lunch. Everyone was quiet and mostly kept to themselves.

After breakfast, I managed to catch up with Lucy in our room. She was folding some clothes, which only made me slightly jealous, considering my paper scrubs. She moved to put on a sweatshirt. As she adjusted her sleeves, I saw white cutting scars and red streaks wrapped around her wrists. The neckline was snug, but there were red marks on her skin there, too.

I wasn't about to ask her anything personal, but I was curious. Had she tried to strangle herself like me? If so, she obviously made a better effort. I don't remember how the conversation started, but she somehow felt comfortable enough sharing with me that her husband had hanged himself and died some time ago. She found his body, and the shock and loss led her into terrible depression. She never disclosed that she had followed in his footsteps, but my suspicions grew, and my heart hurt for her.

Later that day, we did a group activity listening to mainstream music with encouraging lyrics. They were all about persevering through struggle and not giving up. That seemed fitting for a psych ward where most patients had either attempted suicide or seriously considered it. I appreciated the encouragement and accepted it gladly, but wound up thinking more about myself than the music.

I'd tried the whole "positive thinking and clean living" fad. I had been carrying the burden of depression, anxiety, and disorder on my own for seven years. The only place it led me was a pit of despair. Even reaching out for help by going to Dr. Kelly had been the responsible, positive, and right choice; yet here I was voluntarily admitted to the loony bin.

Despite pessimism and realism knocking at the door of my psyche, I chose to continue going through the motions of whatever treatment the hospital deemed necessary. You must find meaningful symbolism in pop music. [Check]. You should eat all of your food at every meal. [Check]. We expect you to attend every group activity and take part willingly. [Check].

If that's what it would take to get some answers after being in the dark so long, I would comply. Maybe that answer would come from a doctor, but perhaps it might come from a nurse, counselor, or fellow patient. I had come too far for this experience not to be life-changing, so I must be open and ready to receive.

The opportunity came for me to make a quick phone call to Victoria, who had returned to the hospital the previous night to find me missing. She was frustrated that nobody from the hospital bothered to update her, but was glad I was safe. She agreed to bring me some toiletries and comfortable clothes.

That same evening, after dinner, she brought my personal items and stayed for a brief visit. My father also came, and it was encouraging to see friendly, familiar faces in such a bizarre place. We talked about the weirdness of it all, and on account of my tiredness, I joked that they must be putting sedatives in the food. Our meeting was short, but energizing. I was excited to get what I needed and get out!

DAY TWO

Finally, it came time for my appointment with one of the hospital's psychiatrists. This was what I'd been looking forward to the most, expecting to receive answers. They told me I would meet the doctor after breakfast that morning. I ate, showered, sat primly on my bed, and readied myself for the doctor to arrive, full of hope and anticipation.

I thrust away an unexpected rush of disappointment the moment he walked in the door. A strange premonition said, "No, this isn't it. It isn't him," but there was no room for such an intrusion. My mind and heart were set on finding a solution, and a random gut feeling was not going to get in the way. This moment was supposed to be pivotal and decisive, but it wasn't. The exchange was brief and anticlimactic. He asked me some basic questions, and we talked about medication.

He didn't seem to be interested in investigating or analyzing anything. He looked at his clipboard filled with papers for much of our time. His conclusion did not include anything I hadn't already figured out myself.

"Obviously, you're depressed, but I think you just need more time on the medication. You aren't hallucinating or hearing voices, so you don't have schizophrenia. You don't have any signs of mania, so we can rule out bipolar disorder, too."

To say I was gutted to hear absolutely no new information or insight from this so-called expert's mouth would be an understatement. This exchange should have changed everything, but it didn't. I had attempted to manifest a breakthrough for myself by expecting everything to be revealed, once and for all, through the limited knowledge and understanding of this mortal man. I was floored and disappointed, confronted by yet another experience of stagnant stillness. He didn't see me, inside or out. He didn't even take the time to look.

I submissively nodded and answered his questions about medication. Then he asked, "So, when were you thinking you wanted to leave?"

Realizing there was nothing left to gain and adapting quickly, "Maybe tomorrow?"

He thought for a moment and agreed. "As long as you keep going to group meetings and take your meds, we can do that. I'll get the paperwork done, and you can be out of here tomorrow." With a thank you and a grim smile, he left, and that was it.

I didn't believe this doctor was ill-meaning or negligent, but surely he had missed something. Despite how crushing that feeling was, the only thing left to do was move on. Sullenly, I made my way to group therapy, remembering the hospital staff's advice: "The more you show willingness to participate, the more we believe you can handle going home."

The group was held in a lounge-type room with couches, chairs, and a large TV. Almost everyone was there, with one counselor to wrangle all our thoughts, emotions, and circumstances into a cohesive lesson for growth. We started with a game of Pictionary to break the ice. It was hardly fun, not at all entertaining, but it did give me time to try to relax.

Eventually, we got down to the nitty-gritty, and the counselor started asking us some deep questions. The chaotic influx of off-topic responses drowned out any memory of the specific questions. Everyone seemed to want to talk about what they were going through, no matter how personal or inappropriate. It was jarring to say the least.

A middle-aged, wheelchair-using amputee woman named Betty spoke at length about all that her abusive father had done to her. She shared these horrific events with little emotion, simply stating the facts. She then talked about all the other ways she'd been victimized in life, specifically and more recently by a boyfriend of some sort.

It was obvious she had been through the wringer more than a few times, but she also played the part of a victim well. She never talked about herself except to explain what someone had done to her. When the counselor tried to redirect and ask her about her own thoughts and actions, she would get irritated and ramble on about something else.

A young man named Benny was much more ordered, but no more self-aware than Betty when sharing his backstory. There was a church shooting, and he had witnessed the horrific carnage. He described bullets and blood everywhere. Seeing people he knew, friends and children, slaughtered and ripped apart. His descriptions were brief and censored enough, but he was much too nonchalant.

There was a look in his eyes that said he was still reliving it. His body language was stiff and choppy. He laughed and smiled more than was appropriate, considering the topic. It was all a defense mechanism. He talked about himself more than Betty and was vocal about his plan to "stay positive" despite these haunting memories. Perhaps he was simply having a good day, and tomorrow might bring more trouble than a positive attitude could fix.

At the close of the second day, my confidence plummeted. Everyone else seemed to have a reason for being so troubled. Benny was lost in trauma, Lucy was lost in despair, and Betty was lost in victimhood. What was I lost in?

I had nothing to name but unexplainable chronic depression. Was there any place for me if it wasn't the psych ward? There was no logical reason my depression should be this debilitating and relentless. It came back repeatedly, no matter the circumstances.

I was desperate to find the root of the problem, certain that there was some underlying cause, yet experts kept telling me all was well. The psychiatrist who was supposed to hold my future in the palm of his hand didn't uncover or release anything.

"The Prozac seems to be working okay. We'll keep you on that, and you should feel better soon," he had said.

Maybe he was right, and this mountain was really a molehill in disguise. Either way, I was ready to move on from this circus.

LAYING IT DOWN AND LETTING GO

Despite the discouragement in my chest, I took a deep breath and released all of my expectations with it. After sitting and thinking for a while, I got off my bed, walked over to the window, and stared out. The last forty-eight hours had contained a lot of staring. Cars drove by, people walked and talked, and planes flew to far-off places. There was nothing else to do but stare at everything I was missing out on.

God gave me the precious gift of life to steward well, but my misguided efforts to do so were unsuccessful. I had failed. I had lost. Did it even matter? I couldn't say, but the part my choices had played was evident. I wasted a lot of time over the years, but thank God I hadn't lost my life completely. For the first time, clarity came to me forty feet above ground, behind glass, completely out of touch and displaced.

This burden was not my parents', siblings', or friends' to carry, but it wasn't mine either. Even though these problems manifested through my own imperfections, no personal attempt at perfection would relieve me from that weight. I understood and believed, from a childhood faith, that Jesus Christ had died for my sins. If He died for my sins, then He had carried this burden long before it existed.

I fought Him, resisted Him, and pulled away for no reason other than to be obstinate. I said "No" repeatedly to His sorrow and my own destruction. I was hurt and mangled and scarred, but there was nothing to blame but my own sense of self-reliance. This was my hour to return to grace. The only thing left to do was to let go. As the book of Matthew says:

> Come to me, all you who are weary and burdened,
> and I will give you rest. Take my yoke upon you
> and learn from me, for I am gentle and humble in heart,
> and you will find rest for your souls.
> For my yoke is easy and my burden is light.
> MATTHEW 11:28–30, NIV

Staring out that hospital window, a silent prayer fell from my lips. "God, I think I'm ready to do it your way now." Warmth spread all over my body from the inside out, and peace filled my heart. With a small smile of submission, I turned away from that window and never looked back.

DAY THREE

The last day of my stay at the hospital left me full of resolution to move on, go home, and get my freedom back. I couldn't wait to leave this place that was stuck in time. I had certainly taken my freedom for granted and was determined to never enter a psych ward again. This was the first and last time. The monotony of sticking to a schedule made for you, but not by you, was tiring and draining.

It was the little things that increasingly bothered me. Not being able to shave my legs or underarms was surprisingly frustrating. Preparing my own meals and eating however much or little I wanted without being subject to speculation felt like a distant memory. Getting woken up at the crack of dawn for bloodwork every morning made me feel like a test subject. The thirty-minute room checks from the nurses were unnecessary, as I was no longer suicidal. It was all getting a little ridiculous. I didn't belong there.

Fortunately, the doctor completed all the paperwork promptly as promised, and my discharge was set for later that afternoon. I packed my few belongings after taking lunch in my room, preparing to leave as soon as possible. I declined to join whatever the group activity was that day and sat at the desk in my room.

They had already agreed to let me leave, so why continue playing the game? It wasn't worth it. Music therapy, group counseling, and sharing personal information hadn't led to any answers, only more questions. Regardless of the underlying bummer, I was free from the burden of needing to know everything. I had surrendered this area to God, and meant it. I was going to let go and let Him carry me forward.

My sister arrived to pick me up, and I was ecstatic to go. Walking out of those doors lifted a lingering weight off my shoulders. I left that hospital not knowing anything new about myself, but feeling so much better. To breathe the polluted city air for the first time in three days was to breathe for the first time ever! Oh, the warmth of the blistering July sun felt marvelous!

As we drove home, I gawked out the window like a child. To see the cars driving by up close, to hear the music on the radio, to be stuck in traffic felt like the biggest blessing. How could I not have seen this beauty before? How could I have ever lost sight of God's grace, which is always sufficient? When we arrived home, I cleaned my room to cement this fresh start.

REFLECTION AND CORRECTION

Surrender is Victory

To surrender is to stop resisting. To surrender *spiritually* is to stop resisting God. He is not an opponent worth fighting against because He never loses!

Whatever battles we face in life, we must remember that God is always with us and for us. The devil, the world, and sin are our enemies. God is not.

He is our greatest ally. Surrendering to Him will always result in victory.

What is a "fight" in your life that has not been fully surrendered to God?

In prayer, surrender this area to Jesus. *Exchange* your heavy burden for a light one and *submit* yourself to God's good and perfect will. Reflect below on what has changed in you because of this surrender:

EXCHANGE:

Come to me, all you who are weary and burdened,
and I will give you rest.
...For my yoke is easy and my burden is light.
MATTHEW 11:28 AND 30, NIV

In the box on the next page, list what you laid down (HEAVY) and what you received in return (LIGHT).

HEAVY	LIGHT
E.g., Depression, anxiety, and failure	E.g., Gratitude, peace, and faith

SUBMIT:

> Father, if you are willing, take this cup from me;
> yet not my will, but yours be done.
> LUKE 22:42, NIV

List previous rebellion in flesh (IN MY WILL) and future submission by spirit (IN GOD'S WILL).

IN MY WILL	IN GOD'S WILL
E.g., Excessively worrying	E.g., Trusting God's sovereignty

CHAPTER 6

True Identity is Found in Christ

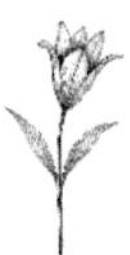

Many doctors relied solely on medicine to treat their psychiatric patients, but Dr. Kelly was not one of them. There was still a clear expectation for the antidepressants to encourage a positive change in me, but they hadn't done so yet. Considering everything, he was wise enough to suspect that factors other than my brain might be contributing to the problem. He recommended cognitive behavioral therapy to help get to the bottom of it all. So, although the hospital did not require it, I started seeing a counselor once a week.

GUIDANCE AND COMFORT

One goal of the therapy was to provide a deeper understanding of any clinically diagnosed conditions. More comprehensive knowledge of said subjects, like anxiety and depression, would help me identify any resulting patterns of thinking and behavior that are harmful. After coming to recognize these unhealthy patterns, I might replace them with healthy alternatives that would change my life for the better. I was open and optimistic about trying out this new tool and eager to gain a confidant.

The counselor's name was Febe, and I liked her right away. Her quiet confidence and obvious compassion for me were a welcome change from the sterile, controlled, and sometimes fearful nature of the physicians I'd encountered. Febe became one of the few people I could be honest and transparent with. Not only was I able to describe the darkness and peril of my depression and anxiety, but I could also reveal pivotal experiences from my childhood and the stresses of growing into adulthood.

It was a relief to let go of pain from the past and from the present. She would ask how everything was going, and I would let her have it without holding back. I might have confided in a friend or mentor before her, but there were none. If my relationship with God were stronger and less neglected, He would have been the best counselor, much better than Febe. However, He would use this setting and strategy as a stepping stone to bring me even closer to Him.

Licensed professional counselors are not allowed to diagnose officially, but that likely didn't stop her from doing so unofficially. With each visit, I became comfortable revealing even more about myself, giving her a new piece to add to the puzzle. I often wasted time blubbering and rambling on, but Febe was gracious and methodical. She allowed me to wallow, even offering tissues, all the while studying these outbursts of sensitivity. After a while, she led me back to the rational path by asking all the right questions.

In true CBT fashion, Febe also called me to action every single week. When I complained about inconsistently completing menial tasks, she instructed me to break up the work and do one thing per day. When I complained of being emotionally exhausted, she encouraged me to journal moments of upset as they happened to avoid bottling up those feelings. These constructive suggestions and Febe's kind personality did their part to get me out of my head and feelings, and onto a sustainable path forward.

A HOPE AND A FUTURE

While devoting myself to therapy, returning to work, and trying hard to be a good steward of God's mercies and blessings, something surprising happened. An acquaintance and coworker named Jose crashed into my life, or rather, I crashed into his. We had met briefly twice, and I'd been wildly attracted to him, but nothing further was pursued. I was too distracted by my mental hauntings, and he by a recent breakup, as would come out later. But when our paths crossed for the third time, we were both emotionally free enough to express interest in getting to know one another.

However, "getting to know one another" quickly turned into "knowing each other very well," and we became inseparable. He lived in a studio apartment that happened to be on my way to work, and it became a place of refuge for me. I took every opportunity to stop by, often packing a small bag to stay overnight. I was so caught up in the excitement of having a special someone that all sense of propriety and morality was abandoned.

Despite the consequences that would inevitably come to us later, Jose was a major positive influence in this new season of my life; I prayed he would be part of my future. He was older and wiser, but not callous. I had never met anyone as kind and understanding. He watered the sprouts of hope that were growing in me.

HOUSE OF MIRRORS

On one such visit to Jose's, I was dreading going to see my new psychiatrist for the first time. Unlike with therapy, it was necessary to agree to this treatment upon discharge from the hospital. Despite agreeing to go, they wouldn't track me down if I bailed, which was becoming a serious consideration. It might be better to skip it and not receive answers than go and be disappointed again. It seemed unnecessary, and I was wary of more medical intervention.

I was still taking the Prozac and doing okay with it, especially being blissfully distracted by Jose. Self-harm and suicidal ideation were temptations of the past. But Jose encouraged me to comply. He rationalized that I couldn't be any worse off since I could take or leave whatever information this new doctor offered. So, with this reminder of my autonomy, I went through with it. After his apartment faded from the rear-view mirror during the short drive, the butterflies in my tummy grew harder to ignore. They weren't sweetly fluttering butterflies, but butterflies beating their wings with ferocious urgency.

I hadn't given the visit too much thought previously, but my expectations were low enough that what transpired would be a tremendous shock. I entered the parking lot surrounded by tall oak trees, parked in the shade, and sat still, preparing myself to go in. The office was one of six large, modern buildings completely covered in mirrors. I didn't know what the original concept or idea was behind this complex full of reflective structures, but I didn't like it. Being forced to look inward and see myself was quickly becoming exhausting.

Lately, I'd found myself caring less about appearances and more about the invisible truth. Maybe it was spiritual discernment preparing me to receive said truth, but I couldn't shake the desire to leave. Circumstances were improving, and I was certainly happier after meeting Jose. Why couldn't I just hide behind him? Why did I have to keep facing these fears? Before panic could set in, a flashback to Jose's reassurance helped calm me down. It wasn't that serious. I could take or leave whatever I wished.

Just go in and get it done, I thought.

I made my way to the second floor, found the correct suite, and entered the busy waiting room. It reminded me of a hotel lobby with fabric couches and armchairs rather than the typical clinic waiting room usually filled with vinyl upholstery. The check-in process for my appointment with Dr. Louis Fabre was quick and painless. This new doctor was completely unknown to me, but that was fine because he would reveal himself shortly. While waiting for my name to be called, I tried to remain unaffected and neutral. Before long, a heavy door opened, and a tall, older gentleman with thinning white hair called, "Elizabeth?"

I got up and followed him a few paces down the hall to his office. He instructed me to close the door rather gruffly and plopped down in his large desk chair. Sitting across from him, I prepared myself to be disappointed or offended, since he seemed even less interested than the doctor at the hospital. He had a tabletop behind him covered with photos of children and grandchildren, which put me at ease a little. His heart couldn't have been completely lost or jaded in his profession if there were people he loved, right?

He started with the question I'd heard over twenty times since first seeking intervention, "Why are you here today?"

I disclosed how I'd dealt with depression for years, but after finally getting on an antidepressant, it got worse. So much worse, I had recently ended up in the hospital for suicidal ideation. Dr. Fabre nodded as I relayed the happenings of the last couple of months, and I could tell his brain was working double-time. Then he asked me another series of questions, some I'd never heard before. While I answered him briefly, my thoughts filled in the gaps more thoroughly.

"Do you often start a project without finishing it?"

"Yes." *Starting was easy, but finishing was impossible.*

"Do you have trouble sleeping at night?"

"Yes." My sleep was disturbed much more often than it was undisturbed.

"Do your thoughts move quickly? At times, uncontrollably?"

"Yes." All the time, it can be deafening.

"Do you sometimes think you're better than others?"

"Yes." There were times when I thought I was the most important person in the world; at other times, I thought I was worthless.

"Do you have any family history of mental illness?"

"Yes." *Immediate and extended family on both sides.*

Dr. Fabre retired his pen and paper and leaned back in the chair to look at me. Then he took a deep breath and started speaking, not about me, but about himself.

"I have been doing this for a long time," Dr. Fabre said. He proceeded to list his professional accomplishments. He was a pioneer in psychiatry. He had spent many years developing drugs and clinically testing their efficacy. He'd also never stopped seeing patients throughout it all, so his experience in diagnosing and treating was superior to that of other physicians.

I had no idea why he was telling me all this until he dropped the bomb that would change my life forever.

"You have bipolar disorder, type II."

He explained that type II differed greatly from type I, which is why everyone else had missed it. Instead of the well-known mania, I had probably experienced the lesser-known *hypo*mania variety, which can be very difficult to recognize.

"Some doctors don't even know there is a type II," he continued, "but I do. And you have it."

I scoffed in disbelief and shook my head as tears filled my eyes. His expression softened as he continued.

"Listen, you are a very beautiful young lady. We're going to find the right medication, and as long as you stay on it, you will live a very happy life."

I wasn't sure what beauty had to do with it, but it was clear he'd broken this kind of news before, with a similar reaction.

Suddenly, my doubt morphed into something akin to fear. The doctor was so certain. But why was he so certain? A sinking feeling grew in my gut as I heard his voice, but no longer registered the words that came out. He wasn't guessing; he *knew*. It was as if this doctor, whom I'd known for five minutes, could read my mind like a map of his hometown. I didn't have time or space to follow these feelings further because his speech became clear again.

He quickly switched from diagnostic mode to treatment mode. He rolled over to his computer and continued speaking to me, making no more eye contact.

"I'm going to start you on lithium," he said.

That certainly rattled me further because I wasn't aware that a drug like lithium was still being prescribed. Images of twentieth-century insane asylums flashed before me. Dr. Fabre continued.

"Along with lithium, we'll do a couple of others [which would be Abilify and Trileptal] to help stabilize your moods and slow down those thoughts. I'd also like to try Wellbutrin, which is a different kind of antidepressant than what you're taking now. It should be better. You'll take those once a day, and then you'll get a sleep aid [Trazodone] and an anti-anxiety medicine [Clonazepam] to use as needed."

It was all happening so fast, I couldn't fully digest that he was prescribing *six* new medications.

He finished his treatment plan with a promise that he would adjust or discontinue any medication if I found the side effects too intense or debilitating. He did not describe what any of those side effects might be, but I agreed, not knowing what else to do. He told me to go to the front desk and schedule a follow-up appointment in one month. Autopilot took over to accomplish this before I left the building and returned to my vehicle.

Part of me was still denying the validity of this diagnosis, yet something else told me he was right. Previous doctors had missed it, *I* had missed it, but it had been hidden in plain sight. Just because I didn't believe it, didn't mean it wasn't true. Plenty of flat-out lies had gotten the better of me before. I certainly couldn't trust myself, and this felt especially true about the doctor, but there was One I could trust, and He was moving all around me.

I had bipolar disorder. It was impossible to ignore or refuse any longer. Sitting in that car, in that parking lot full of mirrors, I was finally humbled enough to see my brokenness clearly. The imperfection that had chased me in anonymity all my life finally had a name: Bipolar Disorder. I broke down and wept in staggering relief.

UNCONDITIONAL LOVE

When my mind and body calmed down enough, I started the car and returned to Jose's apartment. My mind completely zoned out as it swarmed with questions, including whether this diagnosis changed everything or nothing. If I refused the medicine, was I dooming myself to fail spectacularly, live chaotically, or even die prematurely? Or if I submitted to treatment, how on earth could I take six medications, manage their corresponding side effects, and still maintain an image of normalcy among my peers?

In either case, it seemed this diagnosis would rule my life for however long it lasted. For a split second, the lies of the past came creeping back:

- *I am too broken.*
- *I am not good enough.*
- *I am unworthy.*

I always needed extra time to process emotions amid major changes, but this was something that might take even longer, perhaps years. It had been affecting me all the while without my knowledge or understanding. There would be much to learn, undo, and reevaluate.

When my legs took me to Jose's doorstep, he let me in.

"How did it go?" he asked casually.

I silently walked around the small apartment. The questions were still so loud in my brain, unable to produce any coherent reply. Jose sat down at the foot of the bed, and he must have sensed that I wrestled with something because he watched me intently.

Patting the space beside him, he said, "Come over here and sit with me."

He fell to his back and cradled his head in his hands behind him. At his voice, my frenzied trance receded, and I crossed the room. I plopped next to him and copied his position, staring up at the popcorn ceiling.

He peered at me for a moment and then asked, quietly, "What happened?"

I shook my head as tears filled my eyes. The words hadn't come from my mouth yet. I wasn't sure I wanted anyone to find out before I got a handle on it, much less Jose. He said nothing else, patiently waiting. Finally, I sighed.

"I'm bipolar."

Hardly a second passed before he shrugged and replied, "So what?"

It wasn't so much a question that he was *asking*, but a statement he was *declaring*. I had been shocked by Dr. Fabre's diagnosis, but Jose's response to it was electrifying. I bolted up as he strolled to the small kitchen to make some coffee. I watched him under a furrowed brow, half expecting him to climb out the window and make a run for it, but he didn't.

Surely, I thought, *it would concern or at least surprise him, but it seemed like he couldn't care less.* He wasn't worried in the slightest. He glanced up at me briefly, and I searched for pain or fear in his expression, but there was none, nor was there wariness. Even though I felt completely changed by this news, he carried on completely unchanged in his perspective of me. I was taught not to look a gift horse in the mouth, so I didn't push him anymore on the topic.

Jose's undisturbed viewpoint was a gift to accept almost as much as the love he offered with no conditions. My affection and adoration for him then grew tenfold. If this flawed and imperfect man could accept me so easily, imagine the breadth of God's flawless and perfect adoption.

Those two words, "So what," had never been so powerful. I couldn't ignore the painful insight of this diagnosis, but I could trust that what needed to change would, and that the most powerful Love would not be far.

Jose's simple and unbothered words reminded me of one particular Bible passage, which says,

> The LORD himself goes before you and will be with you;
> he will never leave you nor forsake you.
> Do not be afraid; do not be discouraged.
> DEUTERONOMY 31:8, NIV

In the preceding verse, Moses told Joshua to be strong and courageous in the face of the unknown. It seemed like God was telling me the same. I didn't know what the future held for my relationship with Jose or the bipolar diagnosis. Still, I did know God's "promised land" for me was something worth fighting for.

GOD USES EVERYTHING

At the following therapy appointment, I was about to break the news to Febe when she stopped me excitedly.

"You know I'm not allowed to diagnose you, but can I take a guess?" she asked. I agreed, curious, and she declared proudly, "bipolar disorder."

I sighed and confirmed that she was right. While she talked about how this new information would change our sessions, I felt a little defeated. Febe had probably known for weeks, and I had been as blind as a bat.

Her analysis didn't offend me. It was just further confirmation of the truth. I wasn't even close to fully understanding how this would affect my life, and there were still so many questions. But this wouldn't hinder my efforts or discourage me from continuing to improve. I reminded myself that while my acceptance had come slowly, God's victory would be swift—in fact, He had already won.

As I made good on my promise to progress, Febe taught me more about recognizing harmful patterns of thought and behavior, specifically from bipolar. An "all-or-nothing attitude," typical among bipolar patients, was identified in me easily. There were no areas of gray in my mind, only black and white, which regularly led to disproportionate and extreme reactions. I needed either to be a major success or a magnificent failure; mediocrity was not an option.

The disorder was a hard mold to break, but Febe encouraged me to make positive choices little by little until they formed good habits. Instead of perfection, *progress* was the goal, however insignificant it seemed, not unlike how the Bible encourages believers to endure day after day, not through self-confidence, but through faith in the One who sustains us.

> ...being confident of this,
> that he who began a good work in you
> will carry it on to completion until the day of Christ Jesus.
> PHILIPPIANS 1:6, NIV

Febe's new instruction, though secular, was incredibly useful for restoring balance not only in my soul but also in my spirit. As I applied these principles to my life, they helped me distinguish right from wrong more easily, adapt my responses accordingly, and overall grow more intuitive. It drew me closer to clarity and so closer to God's truth. In fact, I started reading my Bible again, albeit sporadically. These simple yet powerful corrections impacted me greatly.

Whenever I was weepy or down, Febe would close her folder of notes, listen to me intently, and prepare to fight off the darkness. In a moment of doubt and weakness, when I used the phrase "I'm bipolar," she corrected me quickly.

"We don't like that language. It's not helpful. Bipolar is something you have, but it's not who you are."

In the dry and jaded world of mental healthcare, counselors have the opportunity to be the light, and Febe certainly reflected rays of truth that God would use for His glory.

MEDICATED AND MISUNDERSTOOD

Dr. Fabre might have been able to see my past and present with clarity, but I wasn't so sure about his prediction for the future.

"As long as you stay on medication, you can live a happy, satisfying, and successful life," he had said.

I never wanted medication, even from the beginning! The threat of medicating was why I shut my mother out for years! Chemical manipulation was partially responsible for this chaotic mess, in fact. I had endured seven years of depression without self-harming or suicidal thoughts, and yet after six weeks on Zoloft, I was ready to attempt!

To say I was angry would be an understatement, but I knew that my anger would do no good in my day-to-day matters. I understood that my disordered mind should be restored, but I lacked the knowledge of how to achieve it. God was guiding, Jose was comforting, and therapy was helping, but everyone seemed adamant that medication was still necessary. As much as I dreaded and hated the idea of taking more pills, no other way forward presented itself. I would try the new medication as a last resort and hope for the best.

I'm uncertain how long the medicine took to kick in, maybe a day or two, but when it did, the side effects hit me like a ton of bricks. Before, I was certain that zombies weren't real, but now I couldn't rule out the possibility that I had become one. My arms and legs were heavy like lead, and every muscle movement felt like shoveling sludge. I was tired. So incredibly tired. The sun was blindingly bright, and the air felt thick, like smoke. My mouth and eyes were as dry as the Sahara Desert. My head ached for days at a time.

Most intensely, though, were the chemical changes in my brain. My thoughts were ridiculously slow, slower than I ever imagined they could be. Whenever I called on my memory to speak, or my will to act, there seemed to be a transmission delay as one would see on the news between live correspondents. Usually, the relevant thoughts came late, but often they wouldn't come at all. It became even easier than before to be a generally quiet person because the effort it took just to think was so grueling.

After a couple of weeks, coworkers and customers started noticing a difference. Friends and close acquaintances would speak to me as normal, then do a double-take and stare at my face, searching my eyes. I knew my pupils had been dilating larger than normal; they were probably more concerned with the slowness of speech, slack expression, and lack of cordiality. The medicine dulled me so that I didn't have the energy for politeness or small talk.

I began to recognize the strange looks more easily as they increased in frequency. So I asked my boss, who was my friend, "Do I look high or something?"

She looked up from her work, gave me a sheepish smile, and said, "Yeah, you do."

She had been a good figure to confide in, so she knew me more than most, but this still surprised me. These side effects were truly intense, but I wasn't aware that their extreme nature was so visible.

"Well, you know I'm not, right?" I continued. "It's just the new medication."

"Yeah, I know. Maybe the dose is too high?" She suggested calmly, but the conversation ended there.

For about a month, the side effects of these new psychiatric drugs held me down. Eventually, they did level out slightly, but I suppose that was just my resilient body adjusting. Dr. Fabre continued gradually increasing the lithium dosage for it to "help the bipolar." Obviously, when the dosage increased, the side effects also did. I coped by drinking a lot of water and sucking on dry mouth lozenges. I also justified his actions, thinking, "He's the expert, I'm not." There was nothing to do but what he told me.

Some months later, after experiencing hand tremors, hair loss, skin discoloration, and relentless body acne, I realized something was wrong. Dr. Fabre agreed that the lithium levels must be too high, but all he did was lower the dosage. That certainly helped some, but my distrust and wariness towards mental health professionals and their methods only increased. Any mental or emotional benefit of the treatment I received was overshadowed by physical and mental torture.

After about a year, I got off the lithium since my bloodwork revealed it wasn't doing any good, after all. To reach a "therapeutic level" of the drug, I would have to tolerate the horrendous reactions, which no longer felt possible. This led me to take some time off from psychiatric medication, find a new healthcare provider, and eventually try some new, less intense drugs.

I tried my best to be a good patient, but despite trying so many medications, the episodes of depression continued. Some might have believed they lessened in severity and length, and maybe that was true, but depression is depression, and it never left. I was considerably, yet numbly, disappointed that all these pills hadn't worked as they'd been advertised to me. Despite all this, I still held onto the hope that a cure was attainable. The only difference between pre-diagnosis Elizabeth and post-diagnosis Elizabeth was my belief that God would have the last word.

REFLECTION AND CORRECTION

True Identity is Found in Christ

God will lead us down paths where a worldly label awaits you at the end, but be cautious!

All labels, even seemingly positive ones, have the power to distort our identity into something God did not intend.

Accomplishments, positions, resumes, and diagnoses do not determine our value in His eyes, because God sees all of us at once, past, present, and future. We must be careful not to reduce or inflate who we are based on what we do.

What part(s) of your identity have you found in the world rather than in Christ?

List three lies you've believed about yourself as a result.

____

____

____

____

As Christ-followers, the Bible sets our standards for truth. Scripture can help us correct the lies that fill the table below.

THE WORLD SAYS:	GOD SAYS:
I am too broken.	I am F________________
I am not good enough.	I have a P ______________
I am unworthy.	I am worth S ____________

If we confess our sins, he is faithful and just
and will ***forgive*** us our sins and purify us
from all unrighteousness.

1 JOHN 1:9, NIV [EMPHASIS ADDED]

For we are God's handiwork,
created in Christ Jesus to do good works,
which God prepared in advance for us to do.

EPHESIANS 2:10, NIV [EMPHASIS ADDED]

This is good, and pleases God our Savior,
who wants all people to be saved
and to come to a knowledge of the truth.
1 TIMOTHY 2:3–4, NIV [EMPHASIS ADDED]

Take some time to fill the left side of the table below with the lies you listed on the previous page; then replace them with God's truth on the right side. Don't forget to cite the Bible verses you found helpful.

THE WORLD SAYS	GOD SAYS

Notice in the example how the correction for "too broken" and "not good enough" isn't "perfect the way I am." And the correction for "unworthy" is not "worthy." Only God is perfect, worthy, and enough. We are not.

It is only through accepting Him as our Lord and Savior that we can attain all the goodness that comes with righteousness. God is the Great "I AM," and we are who we are through Him. We rely daily on the strength of Christ, who died for us to fulfill His great plans and purposes so that, in the end, He receives all credit and glory.

PART THREE:

THE LIGHT

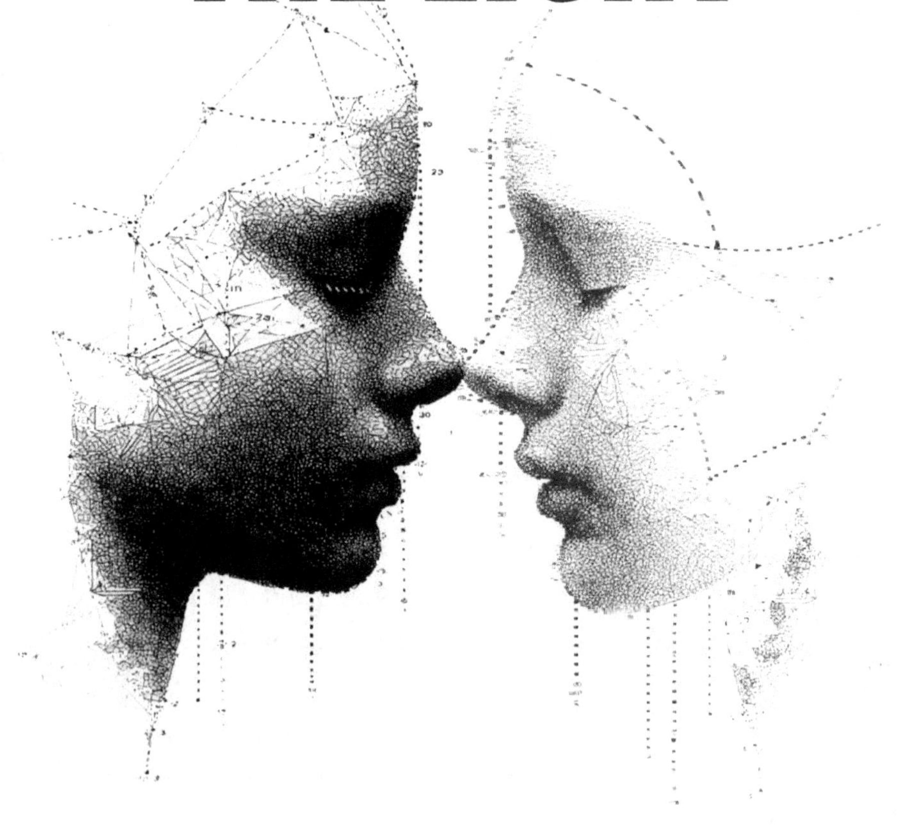

CHAPTER 7

Love is a Choice

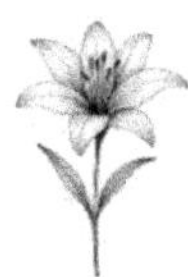

This man, Jose, whom I'd met and quickly fell in love with, owned my heart. Despite the many challenges of accepting and navigating this new diagnosis, I felt lighter.

THE SERIOUSNESS OF LOVE

Jose wasn't afraid of bipolar disorder or its manifestations. He wasn't afraid of me. Like no one else, he saw me clearly through the chaos and nonsense. His slow yet sincere love for me, someone he hardly knew, brightened my outlook on life.

Certainly, he was the one God had promised. The time of waiting on God to reveal my one and only was over! Doubts of a future filled with loneliness and solitude vanished. I could fall asleep at night with excitement for the next day because I would experience Jose's love, in one form or another. It was everything I'd ever dreamed of and more. Yet also less.

We only spent a short time together before he had to leave for USMC (U.S. Marine Corps) boot camp. It was a three-month ordeal, with minimal contact. After that, the possibilities of where he could go with the Marines were vast. There were no conversations about what would become of us when he trooped off. So much was unknown.

Even though our separation was fast approaching, we didn't stop ourselves from falling without caution. I had no idea how it would look, where it would take us, or how long it would be until we'd be reunited for good. It was overwhelming and nerve-wracking, but I clung to the hope of my prayers. I had *found* him! The worst was over because we at least had each other to hold on to.

What I didn't count on was his sudden suggestion one day that maybe there shouldn't be a "we," after all. We were lounging on the couch, but while he traced invisible patterns at the hem of my pants, our eyes never met. He was quiet, way too quiet.

Then he nonchalantly and calmly laid out his thoughts, which included a belief that the relationship would be too difficult to continue. He also stated that it wouldn't be like it is now because he would be gone all the time. And it would be better to end it right there before I got too attached.

Little did he know, I was already quite attached. As attached as a flower to its stem. A flower without its stem can't bloom. It can't grow or multiply. A flower without its stem dies! I was dismayed to discover that he wasn't as desperately in love as I was. It absolutely shocked me that he would want to end things before they even began. A several-week romantic infatuation did not align with my prayers for a husband.

My mind swam through a powerful wave of emotions to reach a life preserver of understanding. If Jose was the one God had promised—in this, I was confident—then there could only be one explanation. He was holding himself back. His words did not match what his heart secretly cried out. He had been rejected and abandoned too many times, and those chains had to be broken. I was his redemption as much as he was mine. We would marry whether he liked it or not.

I grew determined to prove my love for him. Yes, there was an obvious connection, attraction, and feeling between us, but he longed for confirmation that he would be safe with me.

> Dear children, let us not love with words or speech,
> but with actions and in truth.
>
> 1 JOHN 3:18, NIV

Love cannot be made complete without action, and his heart yearned for me to pass the tests of both trial and time.

So, I swallowed the hurt and said, "No."

He glanced at me in a patronizing way, as if bracing for a temper tantrum. He was dating someone eight years his junior with absolutely zero prior romantic experience; he must have thought me a helpless little fool. Even though the agonizing tears flowed in a rush from his rejection, I stayed relatively calm.

"Well," I returned, "I'm sure we don't need to do that. Let's just see where it goes."

I hoped that using the terms "we" and "let's" hadn't slipped his notice. He might have been proficient at cutting ties, but I was not and would rather remain miserably unskilled in the matter. He shook his head doubtfully and pondered my sentiment before letting out a resounding sigh and reluctantly agreeing. I could tell he wasn't all in, but at least another major life crisis had been averted.

SEE YOU LATER

When the day finally came to say goodbye, I was already slipping back into despair. Jose began keeping a respectable distance since our last conversation, so I had seen little of him. He hadn't bothered with respectful distance before, but reality must have sunk in and brought him to his senses. Unfortunately, and painfully, reality had sunk in for me too. We had indulged without abandon, and it made the upcoming separation unbearable.

Without a permanent commitment to each other, we had no business playing with the fire of physical intimacy. Now our souls were tied, and we faced an extremely long and unpredictable hiatus. This was difficult to process and accept, and I couldn't think about it without crying. Falling into depression again became a worry, especially considering Jose's attempt to end the relationship for good. His doubts and defensiveness were deeply distressing.

When I arrived at his apartment to see him for the last time, he came outside to meet me, maintaining his newfound duty to place a barrier between us. He looked tired and preoccupied, but he smiled faintly. He explained that everything had either been packed for storage or given away. This broke through the dam inside me that held back a river of tears.

In an instant, he wrapped me in his arms and held me in my sorrow. Oh, how I wished he didn't have to go! If only things were different and we had more time. It felt like he was being taken away, and I wondered how God could allow such a horrible thing to happen. What failed to register with me at the time was how space is sometimes necessary for two people to grow. Especially when those people had already been unsuccessful at accepting intentional and appropriate limitations.

Tenderly, he soothed and comforted me. He hushed me and whispered, "Everything will be okay."

He didn't try to pacify my intense feelings or deflect any of them coldly. He simply remained steadfast and calm. As I pulled away to look at him, attempting to memorize his face, he wiped away all the tears that had fallen. He was still smiling. For the life of me, I couldn't figure out why and was too distraught to ask.

The love and affection in his eyes, despite being laced with concern, gave me hope. He was the one the Lord had promised me. A belief confirmed in that moment more than ever. There was no definitive understanding that I could wrap my head around, but it was as certain as it could be. In that slice of time and space, there was no shaking the strongest of beliefs that he would be mine, and I would be his. Seeing isn't believing. Believing is seeing.

I asked if he would write to me, and he said he would. Then he ushered me back to my car. After I sat behind the wheel and buckled in, he leaned through the open window and placed one last kiss on my lips. Still, that strange, almost sad smile remained. After watching him leave and close his door, I started my drive home. That revealing smile saturated my thoughts. It dawned on me to describe it as *resolved.*

He believed that moment was our last together, or at least cynically suspected it. He wasn't sure that I'd wait for him as I promised and was determined to have a peaceful conclusion. He resolved to be disappointed. Despite his history of disastrous relationships, I recognized our bond was something worth fighting for. Fortunately for him, I resolved to be hopeful. If it was hope he lacked, then I would hope enough for both of us.

HOLDING ON

No matter what happened, I was determined to make the relationship work. Because I'd already given myself to him physically, in my heart, I belonged to him.

His past was murky, and he was damaged as a result, but I didn't care. I was stuck, yet ironically content to be stuck. If his letters didn't come, I would wait patiently for his return. Nothing else could be done.

In the meantime, persevering through isolated struggles would be challenging enough. His character called me to be stronger. There was slight embarrassment that I had been so emotionally loose, especially with an older and more experienced man. I'd had no thoughts regarding the future, even knowing from the start that he would have to leave. I had been foolish, but now was the time to gain knowledge and wisdom.

To my relief, his letters came. A month had passed with no form of communication, and I missed him terribly. He mostly spoke of his wildly intense military experiences and adapting to the changes they brought. He was always incredibly positive and light despite the adversity surrounding him. Each time one of Jose's letters found me, it shone in my hands as a beacon of hope.

Through the discomfort of change and the tears of missing him, hope for a brighter future grew and grew. Sure, I was down without my love, but not broken. There would be no more breaking for me, not anymore. Strength and bravery must flow from me as they undoubtedly flowed from Jose in his current circumstance. He had redeemed me in more ways than one. I strived to do the same for him.

To gain true wisdom, one must plant oneself beside the waters of wisdom. The human heart is not wise and true by nature, but wicked and deceitful. A holy and pure influence is required for a heart to soften and mature. Although my work performance improved, more insights came to light in therapy, and balanced living became more routine, the most impactful initiative I took was not in action but in stillness.

Without Jose around to distract me, I ran out of excuses not to pursue God. My soul leaned further into the Word and soaked up new insight from online sermons. God had proven His faithfulness to me one too many times. I wanted to be faithful, too. Besides that, I needed Him to help shoulder these unknowns and uncertainties. Surrendering once before had resulted in God answering the prayer of a lifetime.

Assuredly, God could continue to fill the gaps in me if I placed my trust in Him.

LOSING MY GRIP

Three months after Jose's departure, he graduated from boot camp and returned, to my delight and destruction. For whatever reason, even though the spiritual teaching I'd heard was good and from God, it only stuck to the surface. It did not penetrate deep enough to change my behavior.

We continued with the practice of physical intimacy and tethered ourselves more tightly together. Sin is never harmless, but I was too blinded by my hunger for attention for it to be obviously harmful. I was not yet convicted of my sin.

As an act of love to my future husband, I didn't see any issue. Unfortunately, although God had promised us to each other, we hadn't promised ourselves to Him. We acted as though we were married, but of course we weren't. No covenant was made. We were unmarried and therefore officially uncommitted. In the covenant of marriage, God requires not only loyalty between man and wife but also loyalty to Him. Neither of us had yet to show that capability.

So, when Jose left again one month later, the goodbye was harder and even more complicated. I didn't stop crying for two weeks straight. Whimpering and whining consumed my therapy sessions. Instead of Febe passing me one tissue, she handed over the entire box. Gone was thoughtful perception, and back was irrational upheaval. There seemed to be no end to the depth of my heartache. Another period of sorrow and despair had crept back into my life, and it made little sense.

There should have been nothing but happiness knowing I'd found my future mate in Jose. But something was seriously wrong. There was darkness, confusion, and fear again. The only rational verdict seemed to be that, somehow, I'd gotten myself into trouble.

> The heart is deceitful above all things and beyond cure. Who can understand it?
>
> JEREMIAH 17:9, NIV

In my heart, we were married, but in reality, we were not, and I could not reconcile my emotions with that oh-so painful truth.

ANOTHER LEAP OF FAITH

Life carried on. Jose continued with his military training, and I continued working at the craft store. He ended up in Virginia, where most of my extended family lived, including my maternal grandmother. Longing to be closer to Jose, I realized there wasn't a lot keeping me in Texas. My job was entry-level, no plans for education were in place, and my significant other was over a thousand miles away. I wondered if moving could be the next step for me.

The possibility of living with my grandmother was comforting. I'd enjoyed visits with her previously, and since then had wondered about making the arrangement more permanent. If I could find a job in her area, my weekends could be spent with Jose, mere hours away. This could be the start of proving my love and commitment to him and expanding my own horizons, too.

Deciding there was nothing to lose, I sought any necessary conversations to put my plan in motion. Grandma Jane expressed that my company would be welcomed. Uncle Edwin assured me that there was always work to be done at his coffee shop. My parents and Victoria were both surprised and supportive. Finally, I discussed it at length with Jose, who seemed pleased by all the preparations.

Suddenly, amid my excitement, I felt prompted to convey my intentions and leave no room for misunderstanding.

"I won't move my whole life for nothing. I want to marry you, and I need to know if you feel the same."

Quickly, he replied, "Yes, Elizabeth, I want to marry you."

Then he disclosed that he wasn't sure exactly when he'd be ready for marriage, but that he knew I was "the right choice." It wasn't very romantic or hardly an official engagement, but it was the confirmation I required to jump off and dive in.

Within that same month, everything was settled, and my plan was ready to be executed. My little life was packed up, and the twenty-four-hour drive from Texas to Virginia kicked off. It was liberating to say the least. Stagnation and idleness had been the peak of my existence for so long. My capabilities would not be underestimated by myself or others going forward. God was on my side, or more accurately, I was on His.

Somehow, there was reliable transportation, money for gasoline and food, and protection for me, a solo traveler. He deserved all the credit and glory for orchestrating everything just so, but exerting my free will by making such a significant decision felt good. I needed only to trust in His sovereignty and authority to make these actions count.

I arrived to the warmest hug from my beloved grandmother. She looked me up and down with a motherly smile. Her small country house was on the outskirts of a small country town. It was quaint and cozy, with knick-knacks and memorabilia from days past displayed all around. She showed me to my room and left me to sleep.

Upon waking, my uncle had arrived with questions about my work and bipolar disorder, which was not a secret to him. His rapid-fire series of questions went something like this:

"How did you come to reach out for help?"

"The depression wouldn't go away."

"What medications are you taking?"

"Lithium and a slew of others."

"How is bipolar II different from bipolar I?"

"Unlike bipolar I, most all manners of impulsivity, or forms of mania, are restrained to thoughts, not outwardly expressed in action."

"When can you start working?"

"I'd like to take a week off to adjust to the move, but if you need help now."

It was clear he was ready for me to jump into the job, but he was also interested in seeing where that position would lead. He wondered if I would be a reliable worker, if I'd be able to pull my weight without collapsing. But there was clearly a more serious, underlying question beneath them all: Would I let him down?

I hoped not. My work ethic was strong, and instructions had always been easy for me to follow. I was confident in my competency, but I didn't anticipate the emotional turmoil that would be stirred up anew. My unhappiness would, unfortunately, continue to affect my work, and the personal choices I would make would be a key contributor to this ongoing challenge of maintaining consistent contentment.

SUGAR IS SWEET, BUT SALT IS SWEETER

In the beginning, there was cleaning. So much cleaning. It was not only a coffee shop, but a doughnut shop too, which meant it was full of icing and sprinkles. These tiny particles found their way into every corner of that place. So, I swept and scrubbed any nook and cranny my hands could find. It wasn't a coincidence that this new job and new season started with a cleansing. Seasons begin as the last season ends. If I had been more mindful, this significance might not have been lost on me.

My place of employment wasn't alone in its demand to be purified. While I wiped clean counters and tiles, God was showing me that my soul needed cleansing. My engagement in premarital sex was a sin, and He was urging me to repent. He was prodding me to choose a different path. Ironically, with stricter boundaries, I might have found the freedom to love Jose fully. He would have respected me for making such a mature decision.

Unfortunately, I was too rushed to perceive the gravity of the situation. I went through the motions of those menial tasks to earn the responsibility of more important duties. Mopping floors was for chumps; making coffee and serving customers was the real deal, not unlike how I went through the motions of giving myself to Jose so that he might promote me to the position of wife one day. There was no patience or integrity of practice, just a drive to be done.

But even after I moved up the food service ladder, the cleaning didn't stop. At the end of each day, there was a dusting of flour and sugar on the floor to remove. So too, it was with me. At the end of every weekend spent visiting Jose, there was a layer of sin and guilt layered upon the floor of my heart. I repeatedly rejected repentance in the vain pursuit of love and approval. Instead of those, only lust and expectation found me.

A LIGHT IN THE DARKNESS

My grandmother was a good influence during this time. She was a woman of God through and through. Her heritage and personal history of service to the Kingdom of God spoke volumes, but she earned a glowing reputation from me simply by being "Grandma Jane." She listened, encouraged, advised, and loved me in an enormously impactful way.

After attending church together, we discussed the sermon, which led to even deeper discussions about theology and faith. We'd often go out for dinner and examine current interpersonal dilemmas, analyzing the function or dysfunction in our family's and friends' lives. Sometimes, this would lead us to confess our own defects and faults. A wonderful friendship built on respect and compatibility bloomed during those months in Virginia. More times than I can recall, we laughed until we cried.

There was one particularly meaningful, albeit uncomfortable, interaction with her that would be branded in my memory forever. We were in the living room, chatting. She was sitting at her desk, checking her emails, while I was relaxing in the recliner a couple of yards away. I was dressed in sweatpants and a t-shirt, looking pretty drab, waiting to take off for the weekend. She was someone who took great care in her appearance, being from a generation that demanded polished elegance no matter the occasion.

She looked at me with a comical grimace and said, "You're going to see Jose like that?"

"Yeah," I replied, unamused. "Why wouldn't I?"

She sat up in her chair and leaned toward me, then asked with a scoff, "Don't you want to look good for your man? Don't you want to impress him?"

I thought about it and replied half-heartedly, "I guess so."

There was a pause in the exchange as she returned her attention to the computer screen. Then she asked, as if uninterested, "So where do you stay when you go down there, anyway?"

We had gone from talking about something as superficial as clothing preference to something more serious. I hadn't ever spoken with her about sex, but I knew her convictions.

She had been vocal more than once in my presence about the unfortunate decline in sexual purity among young people. She believed in what the Bible taught, that sex is reserved for marriage between one man and one woman only, no exceptions. That was the word, and the word was true. If she found out that I'd already given up my sexual purity, it would expose me to her sharp eye for righteousness. She was a bird of prey ready to strike.

I could tell she was fishing for something and so I chose my response carefully. I stuttered out quietly, "Jose gets me a hotel room." It wasn't an explicit lie, but it wasn't the whole truth, either. The precious detail that we stayed *together* in that room was omitted. I hoped this would knock her off the scent of the trail she'd started down. And if that didn't work, I at least hoped that she'd be unsure enough to drop it.

But Jane Grimes was not one to shy away from conflict or debate. She regularly shared her thoughts candidly and unabashedly, sometimes to the bewilderment of others. I normally found it admirable and amusing, but this time, being the object of her potential verbal lashing, it felt terrifying.

Suddenly, the air became thick and heavy. I couldn't put my finger on it until it was too late. She shoved out of her chair, rushed over, and stood before me at attention. She towered over me and demanded, as I cowered, "Are you sleeping with that man?"

The tears welled up in my eyes, and my heart pounded as I looked away from her. This was all happening so fast; I just couldn't take it.

It felt like a giant stone had been placed in my throat. No words would come out. Probably because I knew there was no acceptable response. There could be no rationalizing or justifying my actions to a woman such as her. Jane Grimes knew right from wrong, absolutely and without doubt. I realized that pretending would not work, and escape was impossible.

The truth had come out, leaving me ashamed, and rightfully so. Perhaps I wasn't as ignorant of my guilt as I'd previously let on.

Then, just as quick and surprising as before, she let out an exasperated sigh as if she had seen this coming a mile away. She firmly grasped my chin from its downcast position and lifted it to meet her eyes. She stared at me with compassion and finality as I stared back with humiliation and defiance. It was vexing that she had called me out on this secret sin.

It made me feel small and weak. I didn't want to hear her confirm that. No doubt she would tell me how stupid I'd been. A line akin to "Why would anyone buy a cow when they can get the milk for free?" was expected.

Instead, she declared with a genuine and otherworldly smile, "Oh, darling. God will forgive you."

Then she kissed me on the forehead, released me, and walked away. She plopped back into her desk chair and was sucked back into the computer screen. The roll and click of her mouse resumed while I sat frozen in shock.

My grandmother's words cut me straight to the heart. If only I hadn't lacked the courage to take her advice of repentance.

The way out, the righteous path forward, was shown to me so clearly in that moment. This verse describes the value of accumulating knowledge and wisdom rather than worldly goods:

> Choose my instruction instead of silver,
> knowledge rather than choice gold,
> for wisdom is more precious than rubies,
> and nothing you desire can compare with her.
>
> PROVERBS 8:10–11, NIV

While I wasn't coveting precious metals or stones, I had still allowed desire to make a fool of me.

TRAPPED AND TRAUMATIZED

After managing to un-paralyze myself, I scurried quickly to my room, closed the door, and crumpled down onto my bed. Sad and angry tears exploded from my eyes and my soul. Here I was in another hole, not one of hopelessness but of sin. The devil had gained a foothold in my life again. I lost count of how many times I'd given myself to a man, whom I loved dearly, but wasn't my husband. This fall from righteousness was a smack in the face.

When staring at the writing on the wall that this was sinful and should be stopped, all I felt was fear. If we were abstinent from the outset, Jose might have respected me and my wishes with minimal resistance. There would have been ample opportunity to lay the firm foundation of emotional and spiritual intimacy that a lasting marriage requires. Instead, I constructed a box of problems and trapped myself inside.

Now there was the expectation of sex, but also a thirst for it that couldn't be explained. Despite knowing it was wrong, the view beyond my body was out of focus and obscured. Sex had been adopted as such a regular practice that it became a fixation. He wanted me, and how could I deny him? Especially while marriage still wasn't guaranteed.

There didn't seem to be any solution to this moral mess that didn't involve a heavy risk of losing him. He was obviously still afraid that I'd leave him like so many others had. He craved an assurance of permanence as much as I did, but I had only provided him with temporary pleasure. Jose's background called for an outpouring of spiritual love, but he only received physical passion.

Though I had taken care of him, encouraged him, and indeed loved him, it was overshadowed and saturated by the sin of lust. Before the confrontation with Grandma Jane, it was unclear and nuanced to me, but that perspective changed quickly. It didn't stop because I never said "No," and that's what made the next season of my life so painful.

God had revealed the truth once again, but I rejected it. The shame from my continued, unrepentant sin overtook me. The one attempt I made to hint at my inner turmoil over the issue led to nothing. I wasn't nearly bold enough to express the truth, and Jose did not have the spiritual ears to hear nor eyes to see. He thought abstaining from premarital sex was nothing more than an old-fashioned tradition. He was truly ignorant, and if ignorance is bliss, he was free to enjoy. Because I fully understood the wrong I indulged in, instead of enjoyment, it only led to feelings of torture.

I became numb and traumatized. The act started feeling like a form of rape. It wasn't desirable to me anymore, but it happened anyway. Of course, Jose had no way of knowing this, as I refrained from refusing or rejecting him. In fact, I forced myself to play along and deflect any concerns he expressed. If it wasn't a physical raping of my body that I experienced, then it was a spiritual raping of my soul.

My *mind* said, "No, this is wrong."

My *emotions* said, "Stop, this is too much."

My *will* so desperately wanted to push him away, but I instead lay frozen.

The more this happened, the more I resorted to my old habit of hiding. This time, instead of hiding symptoms of depression, I hid symptoms of trauma. I couldn't find the strength to stop it all, and therefore, focused on minimizing the damage. I kept the hurt from Jose and bore it on my own. My rationalization told me that this must be the apt punishment for my unrepentant sin.

LEANING ON MY OWN UNDERSTANDING

All that persevering and overcoming in our relationship, but no victory, because I was once again resisting surrender. I failed God's test to lay down every part of my life continuously. A new life season meant another pit of foolishness to fall into. The pessimistic and defeated attitude of my past returned with vigor. God sent this man to be my husband, not a self-indulgent lover. Yet, acting in my flesh, he was accepted and treated as such. In so many ways, God had warned me to guard my heart, but I let it lead me to injury, anyway.

While a sermon's truth resonated with me on Sundays, its practical application was rejected on the other days of the week. If I were Eve in the Garden of Eden, I wouldn't have stopped at one bite of the forbidden fruit. The entire crop would have been gone before any chance of tempting Adam. How could God save one from such desolation of their own doing? He surely didn't want to save someone as short-sighted as me.

Dwelling on costly shame and unrepentance rather than free grace and forgiveness, I started projecting my resentment upon Jose. I called out his spiritual and biblical ignorance while outrightly refusing to practice the spiritual and biblical knowledge I had only recently gained myself. In avoiding repentance, accepting or extending forgiveness became an uphill, losing battle. My heart had been hardened, and, in my eyes, it was his fault for not seeing it despite his blindness.

He could not clearly distinguish left from right, or right from wrong, so I should not have expected him to guide us in these areas successfully. Of course, this was an inadequacy on his part, but it did not excuse or negate any of my own deficiencies. God convicted me with patience and gentleness, and even promised forgiveness, but I allowed pride and bitterness to take hold. I hypocritically dismissed the righteousness He offered and so turned down healing for many years.

Instead of modeling Christ-like behavior, I modeled the ugliness of a wicked heart. This led to my berating Jose for his complacency and indecisiveness towards our future. I figured the only way to right our wrongs was through marriage, so when he displayed caution or wariness, it frustrated me intensely. So much so that I insulted him regularly with false accusations.

"You don't even want to marry me; you're just stringing me along! I have to do everything because I'm the only one who cares about us."

These types of sayings plagued and cursed us. He would reassure me with undeserved patience and gentleness. Occasionally, he would get equally frustrated and shut me out. For three months, my argumentative and erratic behavior steadily increased, and Jose's subsequent reactions intensified.

It got to such a point that one day, over the phone, he asked, "Do you want to break up?"

All I could say was, "I don't know."

REFLECTION AND CORRECTION

Love is a Choice

Contrary to popular belief, love does not come naturally to humans. One must receive it first from God to extend it elsewhere. God is the only source of true love, and to be a vessel for it, we must know Him.

> Love is patient, love is kind. It does not envy,
> it does not boast, it is not proud.
> It does not dishonor others,
> it is not self-seeking, it is not easily angered,
> it keeps no record of wrongs. Love does not delight in evil
> but rejoices with the truth. It always protects, always
> trusts, always hopes, always perseveres.
> Love never fails.
>
> 1 CORINTHIANS 13:4–8A, NIV

The scripture above not only describes the characteristics of love but also the characteristics of God, because they are one and the same.

God is patient and kind. He does not envy what He lacks because He lacks nothing. He is not boastful or proud, rather He humbled Himself to live among us in flesh. He does not dishonor anyone, even those who dishonor Him. He is not self-seeking but desires all to be saved.

He is slow to anger, and in His willingness to forgive, He keeps no record of wrongs. He does not delight in evil but grieves the destruction it sows. He rejoices in the truth and promises justice. His spirit in us always protects, trusts, hopes, and perseveres. He. Never. Fails.

Select the statement that represents true (Godly) love by marking it with an "X."

_____Love is Love
_____God is Love

_____Love is about me
_____Love is about others

_____Love is a feeling
_____Love is a choice

God is love, love is about others, and love is a choice. Choose God and His standards of righteousness, not the world's misinterpretation.

Sex is one topic relevant to love that is wildly misinterpreted by the world. God created sex to be enjoyed, but only in holy matrimony. Any form of sex outside of the biblical definition of marriage is immoral, sinful, and harmful.

Have you experienced sexual sin in your past or present? If so, be honest in detailing how it has affected yourself, others, and your relationship with God.

____

____

____

____

The enemy is empowered by silence. Consider confessing your sin to a trusted friend. In what ways can learning from and sharing these mistakes have a positive impact?

In Prayer:

1. Repent of any sin that has been revealed to you.
2. Thank God for who He is and ask Him to help you be like Him.

CHAPTER 8

God's Design is Perfect

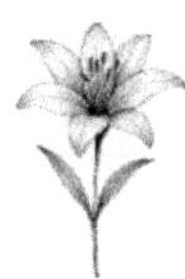

Miraculously, the relationship survived, but our troubles were far from over. There were still many arguments that added to the mess. After Jose was relocated to Washington State, and I remained in Virginia, the pressure to prepare for our union increased. I continued to push Jose harder to prepare for our union. He appeased me with words, but very little action. Ironically, my efforts to pull us together actually pushed us further apart. Not only were we separated physically by 3,000 miles, but our hearts drifted too. He became emotionally inaccessible, and we spoke increasingly less.

HANGING BY A THREAD

As those last few months of long-distance ended, I sank my claws of desperation into Jose with intimidating demands.

"I can't stay here much longer; you have to get me out! I'm ready for you to toughen up and make a move! The waiting is torture. Just tell me when we'll finally be together!"

He always met these confrontations with challenging words of his own. They did not quench the fire of my anger, but they displayed his ability to rise above manipulation and to love me unconditionally. He would tell me how he understood that it was hard for me.

And then he would say, "You don't think it's hard for me, too? "I hate it when you talk to me like that! You have no clue what it takes to be a man. I'm doing the best that I can. We'll be together soon."

By so loudly declaring my needs, I hoped that some kind of manly instinct would propel him to move things along more quickly. But the aggression and intensity behind my declarations only awakened the instinct in him to flee. An enormous pressure to provide was placed on the shoulders of a man who had never provided before. He needed space and patience to learn, yet my criticism and rushed timeline stifled his growth.

My list of expectations, logistically and relationally, was a mile long. His efforts were micromanaged because I didn't believe they could ever reach my impossibly high standards. I wanted him to take responsibility for our broken situation, yet I was unwilling to give him any credit, big or small, when progress was made. My all-or-nothing attitude went to the next level by being projected onto Jose. From what I'd seen, he couldn't do anything right. Not a trace of grace could be found from me then.

Of course, the distance between us was meant for our betterment all along. After proving that I could not be trusted to respect God's physical boundaries by failing to abstain from premarital sex, He forced us apart. It was not meant as a punishment, but an opportunity to lay a stronger foundation. Every season of separation was a shot at redemption for us. I had a lot to learn during both the journey and the waiting period, but I rushed ahead and completely missed the mark.

God intended for me to look inward first, at my own flaws, to be thoroughly prepared for a lifelong partnership. If I'd seen myself through the same critical lens as Jose, my inadequacy would have been easily recognized. Jesus says,

> How can you say to your brother, "Let me take the speck out of your eye," when all the time there is a plank in your own eye?
>
> MATTHEW 7:4, NIV

I belonged on my knees, begging for humility, but I stood tall, staring down condescendingly.

At least Jose was honest about his hesitancy. I claimed to be ready for holy matrimony, yet my idea of marriage was saturated with selfishness. I didn't care about what he got out of the deal, only the affection and attention it would bring me. He was blamed for the pain my folly caused. Through repentance, I might have been healed and restored. Through intercession, Jose might have become spiritually awake and informed. But I could not see past the giant plank of self-righteousness blocking my view of the truth.

HOLY MATRIMONY

Through exasperation and exhaustion, we carried on by the grace of God. I had made it clear to Jose that we must marry, even declaring occasionally that he had no choice. Obviously, he *did* have a choice, and thankfully, he went through with it, despite my disagreeable behavior. Neither the enemies' schemes nor my self-destructive tendencies scared him away.

God knew it would take a special someone to love me, and Jose had the determination and flexibility to fit the bill. He proved his worthiness as a husband daily with undeserved patience and understanding. Although there were those who had given up after withstanding much less, the almost unexplainable love we chose ultimately prevailed with resilience.

Our marriage date was set without the typical fanfare or pageantry. There was no formal engagement besides the prior disclosure of our mutual intention to marry. No proposal, no ring, no man on one knee. Just a conversation about what day would work best to go to the local county courthouse. Jose received some holiday leave around the new year and could meet me in Texas for the ceremony.

After nine challenging months in Virginia, I was anxious to reunite with him for good. I packed up, said goodbye to my grandmother, and once again made the grueling drive. It was bittersweet but also somewhat anticlimactic. One of the most important and memorable events of our lives would be as unadorned as possible. It didn't sit right with me.

There wasn't enough time or money to have a traditional ceremony and reception. I told everyone it didn't bother me, that I didn't want a big wedding anyway, but the sting of loss burned. There wouldn't be a blushing bride in a beautiful white gown surrounded by flowers and greenery. She wouldn't share a first dance with her groom or cut an elegantly decorated cake with him. It wasn't just the appearances I mourned, but the full experience. Would I regret not having the usual marriage memories?

Because it wouldn't look, sound, or feel like a real wedding, I didn't want anyone to attend, even though Jose disagreed. He wanted anyone and everyone there to share in our moment of joy, while my heart was set on just the two of us. I had leaned into insecurity and become quite possessive of him. In my sulking amidst more unmet expectations, I feared irrationally that somehow our love could be stolen.

God, in His faithfulness, ushered in winds of comfort. He knew the longings in my heart and was generous and gracious enough to make the day special by working through others. My mother took me shopping for something white to wear. It wasn't the dress of my dreams, but it suited my personality and the circumstances well. She spared no expense and did her best to ensure my happiness one last time. After being thrust into adulthood, about to be pledged for life at twenty years old, it felt good to be spoiled again.

Jose escorted me to a jewelry store to pick out an engagement ring. It was unorthodox, but no less meaningful. Then, on New Year's Eve, in yet another hotel room, he got down on one knee and officially proposed. He didn't have to ask because everything was already decided, but he did it as a gesture of his love and care for me. That was a moment I'd cherish forever, and it solidified my confidence in him.

Although the process was rushed and constrained thanks to my neuroticism, Jose and I were truly ready to become husband and wife. Submitting to God's will felt like losing at first, but if it meant spending the rest of my life with Jose, then I was happy to lose. Beyond that, I sensed we had won a great battle. There was no worry that day, only anticipation of reaching a new level of love.

My parents attended, along with Jose's mom and one of his sisters. The licensing fee was paid, and we were shown into the courtroom. After the judge arrived, the ceremony began. Jose and I stood before each other, hands and souls bound, as we exchanged our vows of commitment. Under the law and before God, we entered the covenant of holy matrimony. Finally being right with God was such a relief, and I felt empowered as we stepped into our shared destiny. The cords of our souls intertwined.

A HOUSE DIVIDED

The move from Texas to Washington put us to the test. Relocations were notorious for triggering depression and anxiety in me, and this transition was especially stressful. Nothing had been prepared in advance. Our living arrangements had to be sorted out, and I also needed to find a job as soon as possible. Even though God's provision came through quickly, it felt like we had made it by the skin of our teeth. I worried that the rug could be swept out from under us at any moment.

Now sharing our lives completely, we could no longer avoid or compartmentalize the serious underlying dysfunctions in our relationship. Through marriage, we had become one in flesh, but our respective inadequacies divided us. Not a day went by without a misunderstanding or disagreement. Effective and respectful communication skills were sorely lacking in us both.

Instead of basking in newlywed bliss, we bickered like we'd been married forever. He was often away at work, sometimes for weeks on end, which made me bitter. Between our two very demanding jobs and unresolved heart wounds, aggravations that hindered us from meeting each other's needs hid behind every corner. These individual weaknesses prevented us from connecting on a deeper level.

Jose lived by a go-with-the-flow philosophy, while mine was that everything should be planned. If there wasn't a set agenda, our days were sure to end in disaster. I mistook his relaxed and unhurried approach for complacency and indecisiveness, which spurred me to make many "shared" decisions without his input. The more responsibility and authority I seized over our lives, the worse our problems became.

Rather than stepping back and allowing him to grow confidently into this new role, I took over every task and project. *He was never knowledgeable or efficient enough anyway*, which crossed my mind harshly. It was easier to figure it out alone than to silence my hypercritical tongue. In blatant disregard of God's design for my husband to be head of our household, I established myself as a dictator. Jose was dragged further down a path of unfair and nonbiblical madness.

Any conscious attempts by Jose to lead were shut down by me immediately. He did not intend to dominate or demean, but to contribute and provide. Yet I could not allow him to relieve any of the pressures or carry any of the burdens that came with our new life together. Flashbacks to lonely seasons of the past sparked within me a fire of panic. I didn't trust him to take care of us, despite never giving him the chance to.

Through these challenges, God meant to mature my faith by increasing my dependence on Him. By learning to submit myself to my husband, I'd surely also learn to submit myself to God more fully. I should have seen my marriage as a parallel to my relationship with Christ. I hadn't prioritized God in my life, but perhaps connecting through a tangible person could bring me closer. I shouldn't have needed that, yet God, in His relentless pursuit, would use Jose to get me there.

Regrettably, those opportunities were largely wasted. Instead of drawing closer to Christ while discontent, petty conflict was initiated to attract attention. I snapped defensively and proudly at Jose whenever he tried to help. Being alone for so long left me angry and arrogant. Part of me wanted to show him I didn't need his help. It was probably the same part of me that continuously rejected guidance from God.

No matter how much gentleness, patience, and kindness Jose offered me, I was persistently obstinate. My definition of success aligned with the world's, which was to be independent and self-sufficient. I'd never reach that goal if I didn't fight back against Jose's constant attempts to do things for me. How dare he assume that his wife was part of his sense of duty as a man! In my mind, it was impossible for strength and reliance to coexist.

Unfortunately for these twisted ambitions, I wasn't designed to be sovereign over my life or anyone else's. No one is completely autonomous, but women, especially, are assigned as helpers, caregivers, and gap-fillers, submitted to a higher authority. Many times, this higher authority is a husband. Yet even those called to singleness were not designed to be independent, but dependent on the God who created her to be great in Him.

God called me to marriage to teach that dependence, according to God's spiritual order, is, in fact, healthy. By allowing Jose to be my head, I would empower him to be led by Christ. However, instead of encouraging Jose to fulfill his God-given role, I stole every opportunity to exalt myself above him. We would surely be led to destruction if my foolishness persisted.

If a house is divided against itself,
that house cannot stand.
MARK 3:25, NIV

POWER IN THE TONGUE

Even the smallest pushback from Jose resulted in threats, belittlement, and downright hostility. Each time I berated him for something ridiculous or inconsequential, my soul knew it was sinful. Being a born-again Christian, conviction from the Holy Spirit told me my conduct was wrong. There was often a voice that whispered, "Don't do it. You're hurting him." But I did it anyway.

It was clear that Jose was injured by these verbal assaults, but my cravings for control were valued above any underlying sympathy at the time. It was the only way to win this fabricated power struggle. It was the only way to cope with this imaginary oppression. I could not be weak by "letting it go." My options were to remain on top or risk failure, and failure was not an option.

Simultaneously, I understood the inevitable consequences of my actions. If his dejected responses didn't clue me in, my past experiences should have. There was never a more unpopular phrase to me than "sticks and stones may break my bones, but words will never hurt me." Spoken words, especially delivered by familiar tongues, had hurt me too. I remembered my many crying sessions after bearing unkindness from my father, siblings, and friends.

Yet there I was, spewing curses at my precious husband, as the book of James describes.

> With it [our tongues] we bless our Lord and Father, and with it we curse people who are made in the likeness of God. From the same mouth come blessing and cursing. My brothers, these things ought not be so.
>
> JAMES 3:9–10, ESV [EMPHASIS ADDED]

These emasculating and ruthless affronts that I threw around so haphazardly compromised Jose's authority and damaged our bond.

The more I abused, the more God convicted, but instead of focusing on a way forward, I turned back to shame and self-loathing. My frequent thought was that Jose regretted marrying me because I proved to be no better than those who had hurt him before. While it was true that I hadn't abandoned him like the others, he might have found some relief if we had separated. Jose was the man I'd prayed and hoped for my whole life, yet there I was wrecking him instead of cherishing him.

When faced with his hurt, instead of softening it and changing my heart, I shoved the conviction down and justified my sin with lies. I thought to myself, *He needs to toughen up. Challenge is good, and that's what I'm giving him. He'll learn to rise above it.*

This perverse perspective went unchecked for months as I shoved my conviction down lower, deeper.

Jose was certainly challenged, and while he did learn to "toughen up" and "rise above," it was not by my doing. It was God's grace and love that were prayed over him since childhood that strengthened him. A deep determination not to replicate his own abusive father's behavior also sustained him. He took my provocations with courage and dignity, rising above his wife's depravity indeed.

He let me hit him with slander and ridicule repeatedly. In fact, he turned back and forth between his right and left cheeks until his face was stained red with abuse. While I egged him on and pushed every button imaginable, he never gave it back to me, but only every so often. Mostly, he echoed my belittlement with sarcasm.

If I tried to escalate a fight into something physical, he would warn me not to tempt him and walk away. Most admirably, he never held any grudges and never stopped loving me.

SLIPPING AWAY AGAIN

While he endured, I deteriorated. One can only live in a lie for so long without going crazy for the truth. I'd avoided repentance before and had become a professional at it. My lack of familiarity with God led me to see His correction as a threat. I wasn't reading my bible, or going to church, or praying.

I figured He'd always be there and could wait for me a little longer. By exploiting God's grace and forgiveness, my duty to be sanctified only got delayed and denied.

It's no wonder depression, anxiety, and panic returned with a vengeance. An impending sense of doom returned the longer I worked in senior care, which was the first job I had taken after the move. The position was an impactful one and equally rewarding, but the breadth of responsibility took its toll on me. Caring for some of the most vulnerable people came with stakes too high for my low self-esteem to handle.

Families relied on me to be observant, meticulous, and efficient, while their loved ones battled dementia, Alzheimer's, and a plethora of other serious end-of-life conditions. I treated every client with the respect, compassion, and integrity that I would've extended to my own flesh and blood. But, regarding my own care, I pushed away Jose's support and denied myself everything but the bare minimum. After only a few months, burnout found me.

Taking on the pressures of a full-time job and micromanaging at home became an unsustainable endeavor. Finding myself out of my comfort zone at work day after day, then going home to a tumultuous marriage, was more than I could cope with. The problem wasn't incapability—especially if I had relied more on God—but imbalance. This train of obsessive control was bound to crash at any moment because such an unqualified conductor drove it.

Naturally, panic crept its way into my workday. Some days and some clients were easier than others, but the urge to run became increasingly difficult to fight. Despite understanding the importance of my role, even being instructed by God to persevere, I lacked the stamina to push through. If subtraction was necessary for my survival, then this professional pursuit would have to go. So, I took a leave of absence, citing the worsening anxiety.

Letting go of my tendency to overcomplicate things might have worked, too, but that solution hadn't dawned on me yet. The panic wasn't an occupational hazard that I could avoid by quitting. It was a heart issue that required processing.

My leaning towards codependency only intensified without the distraction of work. Every time Jose had to go, my response was fight or flight. Occasionally, I could silence the alarm with a pre-planned diversion. Normally, though, it took a tantrum to expel the overwhelming fear and doubt.

His physical presence had become my lifeline. My mind was flooded with frantic questions and improbable scenarios once his presence was gone.

- *What if he leaves and never returns?*
- *He might crash the car before he arrives.*
- *He might desert me after realizing he never wanted me.*
- *He might die defending his country.*
- *What if he leaves and returns a changed man?*
- *He might find somebody else ... somebody better.*

My habit of controlling every minute detail of our life and relationship had sabotaged my ability to trust him with my safety, and trust God with his.

Jose told me he loved me and would always return to me, but part of me was chained by disbelief. Perhaps this skepticism came from the opinions I previously held about myself. I had been overlooked, ignored, and rejected so many times by so many people. It was never in a loud way, but it affected my self-confidence greatly, nonetheless. I didn't believe myself worthy of attention, reward, or praise. Those lies from my past slithered up again from their dark cave.

I am too broken. I am not good enough. I am unworthy.

It all came to a head one day when I threatened to kill myself by overdose if Jose didn't come home immediately.

When he replied, "We can't keep doing this; my job is on the line," that threat was actualized.

Of course, he came home as soon as possible and thankfully found me only mildly lethargic. He was very upset, scared, and confused. It only drove the wedge further between us.

BREAKTHROUGH BY REFLECTION

My mental instability and confusion had led us to a breaking point. Every little thing led to something bigger. After one too many clashes, a volcano of frustration was ready to erupt. And erupt, it did. There was screaming, crying, and objects thrown around the room. Threats were made on both sides, and insults were hurled back and forth, injuring us both in more ways than one. Desperation for relief fueled the fire, but there was none to be found.

During a stagnant pause, I remember thinking, *Is this how marriage is for everyone?* Ugly and violent altercations like these had turned our relationship into a cold and heartless fight to the death. Each insult was an arrow, and each judgement a bullet. It was clear that if we wanted our marriage to work, then we could not continue down this path of destruction.

I could feel knots in my chest straining to be set free. Not just me, they seemed to be in Jose's chest too. Our hearts were twisted up. Chains of silence had prevented us from being aligned in love and faith. Perhaps if we both committed to an open conversation, we could untangle this mess of lies. The most effective weapon against deception from the enemy is truth from the living God.

His Spirit in me argued that I was not viewing my husband the way He did. God saw the potential for greatness in Jose that I ignored for so long. If I could listen to him intently, perhaps that would shift my perspective of him. Maybe it would soften my heart. My gut told me Jose wouldn't want to talk, but the request came up, anyway.

Miraculously, the floodgates opened, and our tongues were loosened to speak freely. We shared unhindered honesty and vulnerability for the very first time. Jose disclosed his past romantic relationships and the damage he sustained because of their failures. He had never wanted to let them go, but they left, saying he wasn't worth staying for.

Just as I had been told I wasn't good enough, so had he. He did not spare details as he had before. He was completely forthcoming and answered all my questions without hesitation. I shared my years spent in loneliness and how it conceived in me a frantic need for acknowledgment and attention. My desperate prayers for a husband and life-partner also spilled out.

We realized that somehow our preferences, desires, and ambitions had been aligned for quite a while, even before we'd met. It couldn't be a coincidence, luck, or even a point of connection. We had never discussed these topics so deeply. God had prepared us for each other for a very long time indeed.

Our eyes were opened to the obvious fact that we were part of each other's destiny. I was meant for him, and he was meant for me. Although I'd held this belief in my heart like a wish, until that moment, I had received no confirmation from God that it was true. Part of me always wondered if I'd manipulated or forced Jose into marriage, but this experience blew that lie out of the water. God turned the ash from an epic explosion into a beautiful revelation.

REPENTANCE AND RESTORATION

Upon this softening of my heart, conviction found its way inside and upward again. It was painful, undeniable, and unavoidable. I looked at my husband with fresh eyes, knowing things unknown before, and the truth sliced me open. He had been abandoned, overlooked, and mistreated, and instead of showing him he was worth more, I had only affirmed those lies.

Words can't describe how devastated I would be if the tables were turned. He never told me I was too crazy, or too young, or wrong for him. In fact, he had loved me fully and completely despite all the hell I'd put him through.

Feeling his hurt as if it were my own, I held his face in my hands and said, "I am so sorry. I am so sorry."

Some say that the eyes are the windows to the soul, and in Jose's, the negative thoughts and emotions I had perpetuated poured out of them: the pent-up anger and the bitterly swallowed offense in his heart. Faced with the direct result of my actions, I could not continue in the same behavior or posture of heart.

Tears of sorrow streamed down my face for his hurt and my senselessness. I took responsibility for that pain and declared its depravity. I told him I was going to stop this behavior, and that if I ever failed again, he had free rein to hold me accountable. He forgave me, agreed, and we moved forward in renewed love.

REFLECTION AND CORRECTION

God's Design is Perfect

The Bible's definitions of gender, marriage, and spiritual order in the family are clear and specific:

INSTITUTION	SCRIPTURE REFERENCE (ESV)
Gender: Male and female	"...male and female he created them." (GENESIS 1:27B)
Marriage: One man and one woman	"... a man shall...hold fast to his wife, and they shall become one flesh." (GENESIS 2:24)
Spiritual Order: Christ, husband, wife, children	"...husband is the head of the wife, even as Christ is the head of the church..." (EPHESIANS 5:23) "'Honor your father and mother'..." (EPHESIANS 6:2)

The statement "God's design is perfect" does not mean that *we* are perfect because of it. Actually, we are bound to encounter or experience deficiencies in each of these institutions. But God's perfect design is not the problem: Our imperfect, rebellious, and sinful nature is.

What happens when God's original intentions and purposes are abandoned?

- Gender confusion
- Transgenderism
- Same-sex marriage
- Polygamy
- Weak men
- Defiant women
- Foolish children

These sinful deviations lead to harm and separation from God. The bad news is that this ideology is rampant. The good news is that it can be challenged with truth and grace.

How have you rebelled against God's perfect design for your life?

How did it build a wall between yourself and God? How did it harm yourself and others?

The key to success and satisfaction in any of these institutions is individual dependence and reliance on the One who established them. You don't have to be perfect.

Trust in God, who *is* perfect, design and all.

CHAPTER 9

Growth Follows Service and Sacrifice

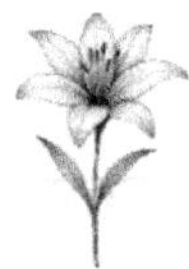

Shortly before we experienced a spiritual breakthrough in our marriage, God sent us word to prepare for another step forward. Jose's father became seriously ill and passed away suddenly. Their relationship had been tumultuous and traumatic, but through a strengthening of faith, my husband was able to let go of his painful past. Even though it was difficult, Jose ultimately forgave his father for abusing and abandoning him and their family.

THE SANCTITY OF LIFE

At his funeral, we received a sign that we should start a family of our own. A minister, whom we'd never met, spoke aloud the name we had reserved for our future son, Geraldo. At that moment, a new direction for our lives became unquestionably clear. From this death, new life would come in the form of a child. It made little sense that we could experience such excitement and joy in this season of tremendous loss and mourning, but we did.

Incredibly, our moment of breakthrough came the very next month when we conceived a child. Even more astonishing, the baby's due date fell on the birthday of his late paternal grandfather. Any doubt we had vanished after this realization. We took it as confirmation that indeed this was a blessing foretold and promised to us by God.

God had already begun healing my and Jose's hearts through our union of marriage. But through parenthood, we would find further healing and redemption.

> Children are a heritage from the Lord,
> offspring a reward from him. Like arrows in the hands of a warrior are children born in one's youth.
>
> PSALM 127:3–4, NIV

I knew clinging to this truth would help me conquer the many challenges and tests ahead.

COMMITTING TO SOMETHING BIGGER

Though the news was not exactly a surprise, I still sat shocked, staring at the positive pregnancy test. At barely twenty-one, I did not feel ready to become a mother. Looking back, there was so much it seemed I hadn't done yet. I'd never travelled outside the United States, attended college, or made any progress on forging a career. The idea tumbled around in my head that somehow this was happening too soon.

The message of modern-day feminism, which says that a woman should not allow anyone or anything to slow her down or hold her back, echoed in my mind and heart. Obviously, bearing, birthing, and caring for a tiny human who would depend completely on his mother for survival would slow me down and hold me back. I realized there would be no stopping this, and the weight of responsibility lay heavily on my shoulders.

Regardless of my reservations, because God had so undeniably preordained this pregnancy, I understood the finality of those double lines on the pregnancy test. It would be as God had said. We would have a child soon, a son, and his name would be Geraldo. While I knew it would be wonderful to have another person to love, the small fear persisted that I'd mess him up along the way. Then I remembered an important verse, which says:

> I can do all this through him who gives me strength.
>
> PHILIPPIANS 4:13, NIV

A PLEASANT SURPRISE

The pregnancy proceeded without incident, apart from relentless nausea, muscle pain, and fatigue. One might assume, given my history, that there would be mental and emotional hardships alongside the physical ones, too. Many women with bipolar disorder report a worsening of symptoms. But miraculously, this was not my experience. Despite the bodily discomfort and unrest, I soon entered a period of mental and spiritual peace.

For the first time in my life, I felt completely normal. There were no symptoms of depression or anxiety, nor did I experience any lack of impulse control. My temperament went from sweet one moment and sour the next, to just sweet. The mood swings that had plagued me and those around me for so long disappeared. I could easily be agreeable, happy, and flexible. Weeks at a time would go by without me even thinking about that thing called bipolar.

Although this was completely wonderful, it was strange and unexplainable. Medication could not have caused this positive change because, to limit the baby's exposure, I was taking *less*! I began to wonder if this possibly meant I wouldn't have to rely on medication forever. It gave me hope that freedom from medical intervention might be possible one day. It filled my heart with promise that perhaps bipolar disorder wasn't incurable, after all. All I could do was wait and see.

In the meantime, everyone and everything benefited from my positive change in attitude and behavior. Adopting bravery and responsibility again, I found another job, and though it could be stressful, it didn't do me in. Tasks were completed with integrity, genuine friendships budded, and whenever something went wrong, I dealt with it and moved on. Resilience seemed to grow in my soul as the baby grew in my womb.

Jose was gone just as often, if not more, than he'd been before, but it was no longer the end of the world to me. There was always a project to prepare for the baby's arrival that kept my mind and heart off missing him. So much joy was found in collecting belongings and creating a space that would reflect how much this little one meant to us. Looking forward in anticipation and excitement wasn't a distraction, but a renewal of purpose in my life.

Whenever minor feelings of sadness or loneliness came, the only remedy needed to overcome them was to stare down at the place where my child was safely hidden. A few taps on my belly would elicit a kick or two from him that reminded me of my newest reason to love fully and freely. Who knew that the two things I'd been toiling to attain for years would instead be given as a gift, if only I'd share my body for a time?

JOY AND AWE

The following summer, our Geraldo was born. The labor and delivery were fast and shocking, but he was healthy, and we were happy. My heart swelled with a new kind of love, and I spent the first week staring in awe at my beautiful boy's face. I fell in love with him in a way I didn't know was possible. It was unbelievable that I'd helped to make something so precious.

Whether accepted or rejected, how blessed are those whom God charges to steward the gift of new life! I welcomed motherhood wholeheartedly at first. I held him, fed him, and changed him throughout the day and night. My heart hurt when he cried, and when he was soothed, my heart warmed. Even in the throes of sleepless newborn chaos, there was bliss.

Our little bundle of joy also enraptured Jose. He'd always longed to be a father and turned out to be quite good at it. Unlike some who take a hands-off approach, he had his hands in just about everything. Not only did he change diapers, prepare bottles, and rock that baby until his arms were numb, but he also sought to build a deeper connection.

The bond between them was instant, because God ordained it to be so. Often, they would stare into each other's eyes as they nuzzled close. He was delighted to be in the presence of his son in every way, even singing special songs in funny voices. Providing, protecting, and caring for this child would be another path to his redemption. He received the chance to be the father he'd always wanted for himself, perhaps an even better one.

PRIORITIES OUT OF ORDER

As our family of two became a family of three, adjusting and adapting became burdensome. My mother instructed me over the phone, "Focus on bonding with your baby!" It was wise advice, but easier said than done. The fog in my brain continued to obsess over everything except bonding with the baby. He was lovingly and happily cared for; however, crucial attachment opportunities were cut short as I remembered all that had to be done.

- Wash, dry, and put away the dishes.
- Wash, dry, fold, and put away the laundry.
- Buy groceries, prep ingredients, and prepare meals.

Apart from these household responsibilities, there was also the new family addition to attend to carefully. He required formula every four hours, even throughout the night, and diaper changes in between. It was constant, never-ending, monotonous work that I could never seem to get ahead of. There was hardly any energy left to take care of my own needs, like showering or helping my body recover from pregnancy and birth. This only pushed me further down a path of no stillness or rest.

I chose housekeeping duties over contact naps, despite receiving soul-feeding comfort from the latter, to lighten my mental load. Instead of cherishing the fleeting preciousness of those first few months, I chased the high of accomplishment. It had been so satisfying in pregnancy to finally achieve goals for myself. I'd ridden the momentum of short-term motivation for nine months, but those nine months were over. Now, I had to give myself up, day after day, for the next eighteen years, to reach a long-term goal. It was daunting.

SOMETHING OLD AND SOMETHING NEW

After Jose went back to work, things at home took an unhappy turn. It became a dreadful struggle to get up at night with the baby. The lack of uninterrupted sleep piled up without relief. Every time he woke up, I cried tears of desperate exhaustion. There was nobody there to give me a break. I couldn't pass him off or tell Jose it was "his turn" because he wasn't there.

Either from lack of support or lack of experience (but probably both), I tumbled down another mountain. After barely 30 days postpartum, depression returned like a nightmare. For every glad and sweet moment, there were two moments of paralyzing numbness. It was not just a slow season, but a heavy one. But because of the overwhelming tiredness, this obvious reality was foolishly ignored and stubbornly denied.

The more I prioritized determined effort over intentional presence, the heavier the burden of motherhood became. And that's how I saw it, as a burden. Challenges and difficulties do not negate blessings; they validate them. Rarely is something worth doing easily done. This wonderful adventure was exactly what I needed to learn true selflessness and discover lasting satisfaction. Instead, it somehow became all about my performance again.

How quickly my perspective had shifted from blessing to curse! My sights were set on reaching the destination rather than enjoying the journey. Babies grow so quickly, and mine was no exception to this rule. I couldn't expect the opportunities to cuddle, caress, and preen a little one to be long-lasting. In the blink of an eye, he would be crawling, walking, and out of my arms forever.

While these sentiments were the last things on my mind, they should have been the first! Unrealistic expectations and imaginary obligations had once again poisoned my ability to see what I was missing, which was a balance between productivity and presence. It took me a while to understand that while time is humanity's greatest resource, it is also a blip in the grand scheme of eternity. What I was doing to survive and to care mattered, but who I was doing it for mattered infinitely more.

This flawed thinking only worsened the feelings of emptiness that accompanied this latest depression trip. It wasn't just emptiness that filled the space between our hurried routine, but also something that I'd only caught glimpses of before. A growing, gnawing detachment from reality revealed itself to me fully and horribly. Frequently, despite the color and matter that occupied the living room, I would stare blankly through it all and wonder, *Where am I?*

The blue armchair, the swirling, floral-patterned rug, and the random yet uniform texture of the walls were all focal points of this delirium. It was understood, in those moments, that I existed as a human being on planet Earth, but even that fact itself became unprovable. There was a serious disconnect between the tangible and intangible. It was confusing, debilitating, and terrifying. Fortunately, throughout these sporadic episodes of madness, there remained three constants that kept my sanity from slipping away completely: God, Motherhood, and Marriage.

Even though the Holy Spirit felt far away (or, rather, buried deep down), of course, He was still there. In this season of weakness, God's strength and care would sustain me. Often, the most difficult challenges present a unique opportunity to mature in Him. He sent a beautiful son not only to sanctify me but also to be a continuous spark of joy. Each cry, gurgle, and coo drew me out of myself and my pain and closer to transformative healing.

Jose was aware of my worsening state of mind and how it threatened to sabotage our hope for harmony. He tried his best to fill the gaps of care and order, but realized that he could only do so much without my cooperation.

Understanding that a long-term solution was necessary, he boldly combatted my denial and hopelessness one day by declaring, "No more. Let's fix this together."

As we talked it through, the clear reality that postpartum depression and psychosis had struck hard became undeniable to me. I felt a split-second of defeat before swallowing it and moving on. Jose's suggestion that we should address it quickly was accepted with no protest from me. After meeting with my doctor, we agreed that increasing the dosage of my antidepressants and mood stabilizer would be appropriate and sensible.

Instead of being upset or angry, I actually felt relieved and rejuvenated. Mental disturbance had once again stolen something precious from me. Not only did it take up valuable time and headspace, but it also started eating away at my ability to connect with the most important people in my life. The bond that I'd developed with my unborn baby hadn't strengthened after his birth, but weakened. It was so devastating that I was ultimately happy to do whatever it took to get to a better place. This tactic might have cut me down in the past, but now I had something bigger to fight for.

After the postpartum hormones leveled out and sleep came in longer stretches, I got to a better place. The depression dulled, anxiety eased, and psychosis lost its grip. Balance and order, or at least a resemblance of them, returned to our home. I let go of my to-do list and held on to dear moments with my baby boy instead. Here, medical intervention had probably been worth it, and I was grateful for its help then.

Although it seemed my hopes for a cure, or even a remission, for now had been dashed, I endeavored to remain optimistic towards the future. If God had brought such clarity and relief in just nine months, imagine what He could do with the rest of my life. My human mind couldn't comprehend how He would do it, but I was confident in my ability to wait patiently for permanent change.

ANOTHER PUZZLE PIECE

In the following months, we made another interesting discovery. A major contributing factor to my mental and emotional problems may have been an underlying physical and physiological condition.

It was hardly noticeable that anything was wrong before pregnancy, but slightly during and especially afterward, it became painfully obvious. Blisters from dyshidrotic eczema covered my hands and fingers. They itched and burned relentlessly. I resorted to wearing gloves when cooking, cleaning, or bathing Geraldo because any contact with the sores was excruciating. Other equally debilitating symptoms included joint swelling and pain, persistent fatigue, and pesky brain fog.

Besides all that, almost every day I found myself kneeling in front of the toilet bowl vomiting violently.

I was worried that the increase in medication dosage was to blame before recalling a memory. One year prior, I'd been introduced to a young woman, also a new mom, who suffered from celiac disease, an autoimmune disorder. The condition triggers a damaging inflammatory response to gluten consumption. She had known nothing about the increasingly common illness until after her first pregnancy. The similarities between our experiences were too striking for me to ignore.

Some at-home research revealed that pregnancy could, in fact, trigger a previously silent genetic predisposition to celiac disease. Believing this to apply perfectly to my current health crisis, I cut out wheat, barley, and rye. Within a week, the inflammation calmed down. Blisters stopped forming, joint pain and fatigue relaxed, and nausea and gastrointestinal discomfort ceased to plague me after meals. Within a month, the brain fog dissipated completely. After three months of avoiding foods that contained gluten, my entire body seemed to function at full capacity, possibly for the first time ever.

Strangely, the physical healing that ensued after cutting gluten from my diet felt uncannily similar to the mental healing I'd encountered while pregnant. God was actively working to give and take away exactly what was needed for me to thrive mentally and physically. Even though depression and psychological imbalance had returned postpartum, I was confident that the battles waged in my body were coming to a close. Surely, the battles in my soul would follow this pattern soon.

This healing strengthened my faith in God's great plan, whatever that might be. It emboldened me to keep searching for more knowledge and even more wisdom to further help and renew my mind. One step of obedience at a time, I submitted myself to marriage and motherhood, and it started paying off remarkably. Yet I couldn't credit myself. Undeterred by my fear and doubt, the Lord had lovingly and carefully orchestrated these things to come about.

COMBATTING DISCONTENTMENT

Apart from these minor improvements and victories, I still struggled to deny my imperfect flesh and allow the Holy Spirit to lead me. This was especially true regarding the unfamiliar territory of motherhood. The worldly standards and expectations of "aiming high" and "finding oneself" haunted me. Being a mom or a homemaker hadn't been an option on career day. It was something that the modern woman considered doing only years after plenty of education, expression, and exploration.

In skipping the popular plans, I found myself in a role typically reserved for those ten to fifteen years older than myself. I didn't regret abstaining from the partying and sleeping around that was so prevalent, but I wondered if I'd trapped myself in a life *without*. Unable to suppress these concerns, they sucked me into them. In pursuit of being something more than "just a mom," I searched for opportunities that would allow me to:

- Contribute financially,
- Occupy an essential role, and
- Experience lasting satisfaction and fulfillment.

Nothing seemed to fit into our schedule or pan out to be worth it, however. If a job compensated well, it needed too much commitment. If the level of engagement were flexible, the little money offered wasn't tempting enough. If both money and time worked to my advantage, the tasks were soul-sucking. It didn't seem to be in the cards for me—rather, in God's plan—to work both inside and outside the home just yet.

Selfishly, I felt disappointed going against the grain of culture as a stay-at-home mom of only twenty-two. There were certainly those who thought it odd, old-fashioned, or even unwise. I felt sad and envious watching people revel in themselves and their ambitions, not knowing if I'd ever accomplish anything greater than motherhood.

My thinking was misguided in three ways. I believed that freedom to self-indulge was the key to contentment. I also felt that raising children was not a valuable, worthwhile endeavor, and that God would trust me with a purpose "greater than motherhood," before realizing that motherhood itself was already an invaluable purpose.

The lies of the enemy fed that selfish inclination in my heart. I learned from the world to downplay, disregard, and even degrade one of the highest spiritual callings, being motherhood. This slander would have been welcomed by humanity's idolatry and greed, just as it was accepted through my failure to follow God's standards. It was not wrong of me to yearn for a higher calling. Still, it was wrong to pursue it at the expense of a preexisting responsibility.

Not obsessing over others' opinions could have helped me realize that my wishes could come true in the very life stage I was attempting to run from. I understood the challenges and demands of motherhood, but it was the holiness of the mission that went unseen. No matter how small, developed, or able, children are image-bearers of God. To care for mine was an assignment I should have been passionately thankful for.

In the spirit of service and sacrifice, we nurture our children and adapt to their continuously changing needs. Each time they fall, we set them back on their feet again. When they ask questions, we answer to the best of our abilities. In moments of sadness, fear, or worry, we comfort them with hope, strength, and wisdom. In the spirit of service and sacrifice, we pour out for our children even when our own cup is empty.

Yet what our heavenly Father does for us, His children, infinitely exceeds earthly parents' dedication. While we mess up repeatedly and need break after break, He parents perfectly and ceaselessly. The point of this is not to provoke feelings of inadequacy, but to encourage an increasing reliance on the One who never fails.

Accepting this truth and remembering my identity in Him pulled me out of the trenches of doubt I'd dug. No more looking for the wrong things in the wrong places or denying the potential of the present moment. Wherever God planned to lead me, I understood that the covenant of my marriage and the stewardship of my home must always come first. A deeper understanding that I ought to be appreciating these gifts struck me hard.

BETTER LATE THAN NEVER

It took roughly eighteen months of motherhood for God's wisdom in this matter to be fully accepted and applied. Despite how long it took, I finally lightened up. Things previously seen as oppressive duties turned into pathways for praise. Instead of complaining about washing the dishes, my soul thanked God for the means to cook a nourishing meal. Instead of rushing through our bedtime routine, I kissed my son's feet, knowing they would never again be that small.

In the past, I might have lashed out at Jose for being away at work, but now I was thankful for being able to connect with him at all. Gratitude overflowed within me for the technology that enabled us to hear each other's voices and see each other's faces, no matter our locations. I praised God for the precious relationships in my life and for His mercies, no matter how small.

Letting go of myself and holding onto Him was what kept me going, even as more challenges came knocking at the door. During my husband's seven-month deployment overseas, it would have been easier to let depression win again, but God's presence strengthened me. I prayed, read His Word, and invited Him into my day.

- In the morning, when I struggled to get out of bed, He was there.
- In the afternoon, when the energy to keep going waned, He was there.
- In the evening, when I lay down alone, exhausted yet sleepless, He was there.

His grace comforted me, and His rule over my life brought peace. The lessons learned throughout the years had finally stuck. My faith matured enough to tolerate anxious responses in my body without allowing them to penetrate my soul. Earnest surrender consistently allowed me to let go of anything beyond my ability to influence. The same was true for depression. It curled up inside me again, cold and dark, but I chose the joy of the Lord anyway.

His guidance shone through the supernatural help that I called on daily to combat old feelings of hopelessness and doubt. His provision was showcased in the home of my brother and sister-in-law, who took us in while Jose was away. His protection was displayed through the scripture written on my heart and prayed over my family. Being led by the Holy Spirit, I gained the discipline and self-control to remain obedient, even through considerable suffering.

Through it all, God was there, being good and doing good.

And we know that in all things God works for the good of
those who love him, who have been called
according to his purpose.

ROMANS 8:28, NIV

REFLECTION AND CORRECTION

Growth Follows Service and Sacrifice

The wisdom of the world says that to experience personal growth, one must look inward (serve self) and up (accumulate).

The wisdom of the Word says that to experience personal growth, one must look outward (serve others) and down (sacrifice).

The book of Ruth tells the story of a young widow and her mother-in-law, Naomi. Despite many hardships and challenges, Ruth continuously served Naomi rather than herself.

> "I've been told all about what you have done for your mother-in-law since the death of your husband—how you left your father and mother and your homeland and came to live with a people you did not know before ..."
>
> RUTH 2:11, NIV

Prayerfully looking outward at the people in your life, who is God calling you to serve? (E.g., spouse, children, parents, relatives, friends, strangers.)

____

____

____

How far are you willing to go to serve them right now? In the future?

How would this service glorify God and strengthen your relationship with Him? How would it strengthen your relationships with others?

In the first book of Samuel, a woman named Hannah, who is barren, petitions God to bless her womb with a son. She also promises to release that same son back to God should He choose to answer her prayers.

...and she said to him, "Pardon me, my lord.
As surely as you live, I am the woman
who stood here beside you praying to the LORD.
I prayed for this child, and the LORD
has granted me what I asked of him.
So now I give him to the LORD.
For his whole life he will be given over to the LORD."
1 SAMUEL 1:26–28A, NIV

Prayerfully and in humility, what is God calling you to sacrifice? (E.g., time, money, desire, comfort, ambition, social media.)

How much are you willing to sacrifice right now? In the future?

How would this sacrifice glorify God and strengthen your relationship with him? How would it strengthen your relationships with others?

While Ruth and Hannah are great biblical examples of how we should serve and sacrifice, Jesus is an even greater example. In fact, He's the greatest. His sole purpose for coming to earth was to serve others and sacrifice his life for humanity.

Matthew confirms this by saying,

> ...just as the Son of Man did not come to be served,
> but to serve, and to give his life as a ransom for many.
>
> MATTHEW 20:28, NIV

The preceding verses explain our role as followers of Jesus.

> ...Instead, whoever wants to become great among you
> must be your servant, and whoever wants to be first
> must be your slave...
>
> MATTHEW 20:26–27, NIV

Contrary to the Bible's instruction, in what ways have you been a servant of your sin? In what ways have you been a slave to the world? (Consider looking back on previous *Reflections and Corrections* sections.)

How did those seasons hinder your personal and spiritual growth?

Personal and spiritual growth that lasts, with greatness and maturity, will only come to those who serve selflessly and sacrifice humbly in pursuit of the heart of Christ.

It is because He loved that we can love; because He served that we can serve; and because He sacrificed that we can sacrifice.

Thank God for what He has done and is doing in your life!

EPILOGUE

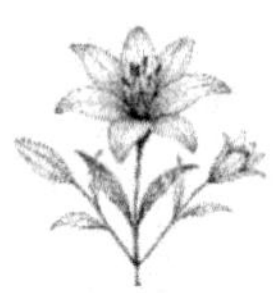

One evening, three months into that seven-month deployment, I sat on another borrowed bed, staring out another window. Of course, it wasn't a hospital bed (*never again*), but I *was* mildly depressed. Geraldo and I were staying in my brother's house, thankful for the comfort but yearning for home. Home was no specific location other than wherever Jose was, and he was obviously absent.

While my husband was positioned 6,000 miles away in Japan, I still lived for him each day. Often, this looked like cooking his favorite meals, singing his favorite songs, and wearing the clothing he left behind. All this was done in an effort to feel closer to him, and to lessen the distance between us that only time could seal in the end. No matter what I tried to dull the pain, nothing could banish it entirely. Wives *should* miss their husbands, and I did so wholeheartedly.

I wasn't alone, but that knowledge didn't stop me from feeling lonely. My heart and body yearned to be close to Jose. His absence left a cavernous void. We tried to speak over the phone at least once a day, despite the seventeen-hour time difference making it quite difficult. Yet those conversations were only so fulfilling. There were only so many ways to replay our days and thoughts to each other, especially while attempting to avoid the subject of our mutual unhappiness.

Caring for Geraldo eased my heartache, and I eased his. As much as an eighteen-month-old could, he took his father's place as my rock. Still, he missed his daddy terribly, and it showed through afternoon tantrums and bedtime tears. I tried my best to be strong for our son, snuggling him, holding his hand, and kissing his booboos. He continued to pull me out of myself and back to reality, as sad and forlorn as reality was.

We took long walks along the beach, digging our toes in the sand step after step, then rinsing them clean in the icy foaming tide. Often, while Geraldo played, I'd sit and stare out at the sun hanging over the Pacific, imagining Jose doing the same. He felt closest there because it was the last physical obstacle between us. If only my hand could reach across the waters to meet his! Then we'd touch again, and everything would be okay.

As I lamented the loss of Jose's attention and affection, God lamented the loss of mine. Every time I avoided, ignored, and rejected Him it hurt and grieved His heart. How often had I held myself back from Him, so close yet so far? Waiting for my husband's return was just now teaching me patience, while God had waited patiently for me all along. Suddenly, my eyes were opened to see God's love through a wider lens.

My pensive gaze through the window that night broke away to land in front of me, where a journal lay, hardly used. In it were a few pages filled with notes from sporadic Bible studies, but instead of revisiting those, I turned to a blank page. Pen in hand, my thoughts spilled out and broke free. They found their places alongside a stray tear or two.

- How can I stay in love with someone I rarely see or talk to?
- Geraldo feels abandoned, and I feel abandoned.
- Jose might be part of God's plan, but he isn't the end of it.

I loved being a wife and adored being a mother. At God's direction, these roles brought purpose and hope into my barren and joyless life. I was endlessly and truly thankful, but wondered again if there might be something more—old ideas of resuming school, starting a business, or dedicating myself to some charitable cause returned. But as I leaned further into my own understanding, the overwhelming sadness intensified.

If these feelings dragged on without guidance from God, they would offer nothing of lasting value. After so long, these attempts to attain something beyond what marriage and parenthood could fulfill stalled. I questioned the meaning behind my suffering, confusion, and perseverance through it all.

What else do God's plans include for me? Which path does He want me to choose? Why would God heal and transform me if not to use me?

There I was, trying to figure everything out again. Finding an answer only required my surrender, just as before. I needed only to ask Him who heard my every thought, felt my every feeling, and wrote all my days in His book before even one came to be. If He was trustworthy four years ago at the edge of disaster, He was trustworthy here at the edge of my destiny.

I wised up, closed my eyes, and prayed.

"Heavenly Father, I thank you for all that you've done for me. You are my Lord and Savior. I am lost again. What do *you* want me to do next?"

It was in that precious next moment that a calling would extend itself down from Heaven. I heard the voice of God for the very first time say, "Write the book."

In shocked silence, I froze, and doubt rippled through me. The voice was again loud and clear. "Write the book."

Relief and awe flooded me as tears streamed in flowing rivers of something unexplainable. The God of all things had spoken to *me*. I'd talked to Him so many times since early childhood, but never had I heard Him talk back! He had chosen to reach out to me in a moment of despair, like countless others, yet uniquely. I'd finally left space for Him to lead my response. There was no demanding, blaming, or interrogating. I simply expressed my desire to receive direction, and "Write the book" was His instruction.

Excitedly transcribing those three wonderful words in the middle of yet another empty page, my heart beat wildly. He had given me an answer. This was the purpose I'd been waiting for, yet a new question arose. *"What would it take from me?"* God meant for me to write my story, but there was a deeper meaning still beyond me. I would soon discover that "my story" would not be a book about me, but a book about Him.

While picturing myself crossing the finish line, I was really at the start. He would continue to challenge and stretch me beyond my imagination, and definitely beyond my comfort zone. Over the next few months, big changes would kick-start God's preparations for a bold future. By saying "yes" to this charge, I unknowingly agreed to be pushed towards greater depths of healing, endurance, and faith.

Perhaps the most noteworthy and miraculous example of God's healing hand would be the fact that I got off all psychiatric medication overnight. It was unexpected, unplanned, and the idea of relapse terrified me. But relapse never came.

Depression never returned, anxiety ceased to cripple, and bipolar disorder faded into the background. Fear of relapse was replaced with astonishment at achieving a state of remission. Previously impossible remission became my renewed reality.

Depending less on the world and on myself allowed me to develop a greater reliance on God and His Word. The answers to my troubles and miseries were hiding in plain sight, between the covers of my childhood Bible. I embraced scriptures like the one on the following page:

But he said to me, "My grace is sufficient for you,
for my power is made perfect in weakness."
Therefore I will boast all the more gladly
about my weaknesses,
so that Christ's power may rest on me."
2 CORINTHIANS 12:9, NIV

I learned to remember Christ's sacrifice and reflect on its impact every day to ground me in truth and grace. In the future, when the darkness threatened to regroup, my faith in the Light of the World was my rock. Rather than fighting tooth and nail as a one-man army, I surrendered each battle at the foot of the cross. And whenever seasons of light shone down on my family and me, we remained steadfast and obedient, refusing to lose sight of the One responsible for its emission.

ABOUT THE AUTHOR

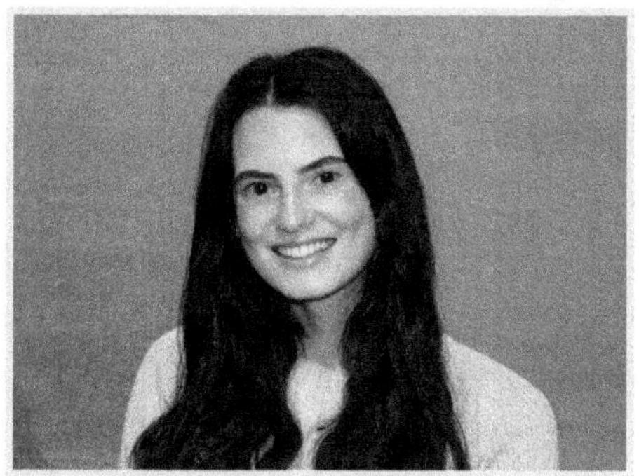

Elizabeth Arce (AHR-seh) is a devoted Christian, wife, and mother. She spends her time nurturing a wholehearted relationship with Christ, serving and being served in marriage, and tirelessly wrangling children, related and unrelated.

At 26 years old, *One of Two Ways* is her first published work as an author. When she is not speaking about her experiences detailed in this book, you can find her serving in Kids', Women's, Worship, and Foster Care Ministries at her local church.

She lives in Texas with her husband, son, and two dogs.

Follow Elizabeth on Instagram through balance_in_him.

www.ingramcontent.com/pod-product-compliance
Lightning Source LLC
LaVergne TN
LVHW020716110826
845149LV00012B/2288